Cultivating Compassion in Health and Social Care

Compassion in healthcare is simultaneously a professional practice and a personal response to the suffering of strangers that is shaped by life experience and a shared evolutionary past. This foundational text draws on insights from Gilbert's body of work on compassion and brings them together with research findings by experts in healthcare to explore the nature and function of compassion in this particular context.

The particularities of empathy and compassion and the challenges of both practices are considered. The process of emotional co-regulation that has a practical basis rooted in communication is framed as key to the experience of compassion. Mindfulness is presented as a way of establishing an attuned self-awareness as the foundation for self-care, as well as for states of healthy connection with patients and colleagues. The cognitive therapy model is introduced as one way of organising the salient features of compassionate practice. Suggestions are made for cultivating compassion in health and social care at individual, team and organisational levels.

This book is essential reading for all healthcare workers and students of medicine, nursing, the allied healthcare professions, psychology and healthcare management.

Linda Fisher is a Chartered Psychologist and has a PhD in Psychology applied to Medicine. She has trained and worked as a nurse, CBT therapist and mindfulness teacher in the NHS in the UK. She lives in British Columbia, Canada.

Cultivating Compassion in Health and Social Care

Psychological and Practical Perspectives

Linda Fisher

Routledge
Taylor & Francis Group

LONDON AND NEW YORK

First published 2026
by Routledge
4 Park Square, Milton Park, Abingdon, Oxon OX14 4RN

and by Routledge
605 Third Avenue, New York, NY 10158

Routledge is an imprint of the Taylor & Francis Group, an informa business

© 2026 Linda Fisher

British Library Cataloguing-in-Publication Data
A catalogue record for this book is available from the British Library

ISBN: 9781032547312 (hbk)
ISBN: 9781032547305 (pbk)
ISBN: 9781003427247 (ebk)

DOI: 10.4324/9781003427247

Typeset in Optima
by codeMantra

Contents

Contents

Acknowledgments

With grateful thanks to my family, colleagues, patients, and teachers of all kinds, who helped make this book possible.

1 Celebrating and renewing the commitment to compassion in health and social care

This opening chapter speaks to the many acts of compassion that flow through diverse healthcare systems on a daily basis. It also urges a reinvigorated focus on compassion, one that consolidates the position of compassion as an essential quality of care and one that is better able to illuminate the factors responsible when compassion is lacking. Finally, the chapter sets out the approach and direction of the book.

The centrality of compassion to healthcare

There is an abundance of compassion provided on a daily basis across healthcare systems world-wide. This is something that is recognised and celebrated by patients or service users and those who are close to them, as well as healthcare workers across the globe. Compassion at all levels within healthcare is as essential to a positive patient experience, patient safety and good outcomes as it is for the well-being of healthcare professionals (Bramley & Matiti, 2014; Durkin et al., 2019; Trzeciak & Mazzarelli, 2019; West, 2021). Furthermore, the well-being of the workforce in itself is also known to be important for patient safety and outcomes (see Hall et al., 2016, for a systematic review). There is also an expectation that all patient-facing staff will approach patients with compassion, including those in non-clinical roles, for example, portering and domestic staff in the UK (National Institute for Health and Social Care Excellence, 2021).

It is a rarity for anyone to embark on a career in health care intending to do anything other than to contribute to exemplary patient care and work well and enjoyably with colleagues. No one doubts that compassion is important, and many healthcare workers feel this as a heartfelt commitment in the work that they do (Dixon-Woods et al., 2014). Patients are deeply appreciative when they receive compassionate care and often express this gratitude directly to those who have cared for them.

It is also the case, however, that a lack of compassionate care or a paucity of related qualities of care, for example, dignity and kindness, not infrequently feature in complaints made to health and social

DOI: 10.4324/9781003427247-1

care organisations. Over recent decades, several high-profile failures of care in the UK have also been heavily textured with something characterised as a lack of compassionate care (e.g., Department of Health, 2012; Kirkup, 2022) and compassionate care has also been found to be dismally lacking in the US healthcare system too (Lown et al., 2011). Whilst catastrophic failures of care always result from a complex interaction of factors, a lack of compassion is also always reported as one of those factors, and this finding alone seems to demand that compassion as an essential quality of care deserves a continued focus. Experts have suggested that preventing unnecessary harms to patients should be addressed as urgently as reducing human error in the aviation industry (Kapur et al., 2016), whilst others have called for a 'reinvestment in compassion as a foundational approach to health' (Galea, 2020, p. 1898).

In particular, for healthcare staff, increasing enjoyment and replenishment in relation to practising compassion is important given that recruitment and retention are problematic in frontline healthcare workers the world over, where it also appears to be the case that morale has never been lower (Banfield-Nwachi, 2023; Bucceri Androus, 2023; Palmer & Rolewicz, 2022). Providing the conditions within healthcare systems for healthcare workers to provide compassionate care has never been more pressing (Howick et al., 2024; Thienprayoon et al., 2022). Compassion in healthcare is a collective responsibility and the book speaks to the need for organisations to take the necessary steps to re-prioritise compassion as an essential quality of care that, when allowed to flourish, benefits both patients and healthcare personnel.

Focus box 1.1   The importance of compassion in healthcare

Patients regard it as a highly valued quality of care
It is important for patient safety and good health outcomes
It is important for the well-being of the workforce
It is repeatedly cited as a quality of care that is missing in healthcare in complaints and high-profile investigations in to harms caused to patients

---

The content of this book

Compassion in health and social care is simultaneously a professional practice and an individual response to the suffering of strangers that is shaped by life experience and a shared evolutionary past. The text draws on insights from Professor Paul Gilbert's body of work on compassion combined with findings from experts in the field of compassion in healthcare and uses Professor Stephen Porges's description of the function of compassion to explore the nature and practice of compassion in contemporary healthcare settings. In particular, this perspective contributes to a more precise articulation of the relational dimension of compassion that has been identified as critical to patients in much of the work by others (e.g., Halifax, 2012; Lown, 2016; Patel et al., 2019; Sinclair et al., 2016). Whilst the book has an individual focus, barriers to compassion, both individual and organisational are outlined.

The text looks to the work of Gilbert, who has demonstrated that compassion is an evolved psychosocial process and explains the use of emotional co-regulation for creating safe relationships as an essential pre-cursor to compassion. Porges's description of the function of compassion is used to understand how healthcare professionals have a role in the emotional co-regulation of states of health-related fear and shame in their patients, and qualitative research reports from patients are also viewed from this perspective. Verbal and non-verbal communication is presented as the nuanced means by which emotional co-regulation takes place. The structure of the cognitive therapy model and the experiential use of mindfulness are introduced and presented as combined methods of attunement to one's inner experience and ways of supporting emotional self-regulation. They also support sensitivivity and a care-filled awareness of, and response to, the emotional co-regulation needs of patients as they arise, and as the basis for healthy states of connection with colleagues. The text gives consideration to empathic concern and compassion as professional practices and considers attitudes helpful for the reliable expression of compassion when it is needed. The text makes suggestions about a revised definition of compassion for use in healthcare that includes relational skills for emotional co-regulation, as well as any other profession-specific competencies necessary for the care of patients. Finally, the text makes some suggestions about how interest in the science and practice of compassion might be grown across healthcare organisations.

Using this book

The term patient can be used interchangeably with care home resident, service user or client, but it is also intended to be inclusive of relatives, partners and friends who may also be in contact with healthcare professionals when someone they care about is unwell or being cared for by others. The term healthcare worker may also be used interchangeably with all other titles describing people who care for others, although it is acknowledged that some healthcare workers will have professional training and others will not.

It is intended that this book further supports and contributes to the ongoing discourse around compassion within healthcare. This is a discourse that needs to be 'held' with honesty and integrity but also with care and without blame, since the analysis of compassion in this text is one that goes to the heart of what it is to be human. The text sets out the emerging science base and practice of compassion in a way that is relevant to all who work in health and social care. Each chapter has one or more focus boxes within it that are intended to draw attention to important information within the chapter, and each concludes with summary points to draw the chapter to a close.

The text can be used in a flexible way, either as a 'stand-alone' resource or used in combination with other materials to increase knowledge, skills and curiosity about compassion. The content of a single focus box or a single summary point, or alternatively an entire chapter, can be used as the basis for teaching or to inform discussion focused on the function of compassion and the role of the healthcare worker in health and social care.

References

Banfield-Nwachi, M. (2023, November 12). *Doctors plan to leave NHS in growing numbers due to burnout, GMC warns.* https://www.theguardian.com/society/2023/nov/12/doctors-plan-to-leave-nhs-in-growing-numbers-due-to-burnout-gmc-warns#:~:text=A%20growing%20number%20of%20doctors,may%20have%20come%20too%20late.

Bramley, L., & Matiti, M. (2014). How does it really feel to be in my shoes? Patients' experiences of compassion within nursing care and their perceptions of developing compassionate nurses. *Journal of Clinical Nursing, 23*(19–20), 2790–2799. https://doi.org/10.1111/jocn.12537

Bucceri Androus, A. (2023, September 28). *The (not so) great escape. Why new nurses are leaving the profession.* https://www.registerednursing.org/articles/why-new-nurses-leaving-profession/

Department of Health. (2012). *Transforming care: A national response to Winterbourne View Hospital: Department of Health Review Final Report.* https://www.gov.uk/government/publications/winterbourne-view-hospital-department-of-health-review-and-response

Dixon-Woods, M., Baker, R., Charles, K., Dawson, J., Jerzembek, G., Martin, G., McCarthy, I., McKee, L., Minion, J., Ozieranski, P., Willars, J., Wilkie, P., & West, M. (2014). Culture and behaviour in the English National Health Service: Overview of lessons from a large multimethod study. *BMJ Quality and Safety, 23*(2), 106–115. http://doi.org/10.1136/bmjqs-2013-001947

Durkin, J., Usher, K., & Jackson, D. (2019). Embodying compassion: A systematic review of the views of nurses and patients. *Journal of Clinical Nursing, 28*(9–10), 1380–1392. https://doi.org/10.1111/jocn.14722

Galea, S. (2020). Compassion in a time of COVID-19. *The Lancet, 395*(10241), 1897–1898. http://dx.doi.org/10.1016/S0140-6736(20)31202-2

Halifax, J. (2012). A heuristic model of enactive compassion. In *Current Opinion in Supportive and Palliative Care* (Vol. 6, Issue 2, pp. 228–235). https://doi.org/10.1097/SPC.0b013e3283530fbe

Hall, L. H., Johnson, J., Watt, I., Tsipa, A., & O'Connor, D. B. (2016). Healthcare staff wellbeing, burnout, and patient safety: A systematic review. *PLoS ONE, 11*(7), 1–12. https://doi.org/10.1371/journal.pone.0159015

Howick, J., de Zulueta, P., & Gray, M. (2024). Beyond empathy training for practitioners: Cultivating empathic healthcare systems and leadership. In *Journal of Evaluation in Clinical Practice* (Vol. 30, Issue 4, pp. 548–558). John Wiley and Sons Inc. https://doi.org/10.1111/jep.13970

Kapur, N., Parand, A., Soukup, T., Reader, T., & Sevdalis, N. (2016). Aviation and healthcare: a comparative review with implications for patient safety. *JRSM Open, 7*(1), 205427041561654. https://doi.org/10.1177/2054270415616548

Kirkup, B. (2022). *Reading the signals. Maternity and neonatal services in East Kent - the report of the independent investigation.* https://www.gov.uk/government/publications/maternity-and-neonatal-services-in-east-kent-reading-the-signals-report

Lown, B. A. (2016). A social neuroscience-informed model for teaching and practising compassion in health care. *Medical Education, 50*(3), 332–342. https://doi.org/10.1111/medu.12926

Lown, B. A., Rosen, J., & Marttila, J. (2011). An agenda for improving compassionate care: A survey shows about half of patients say such care is missing. *Health Affairs, 30*(9), 1772–1778. https://doi.org/10.1377/hlthaff.2011.0539

National Institute for Health and Social Care Excellence. (2021, June 21). *Clinical Guideline 138. Patient experience in adult NHS services: improving the experience of care for people using adult NHS services for the patient.* NICE Guideline 138 Experience Which Outlines the General Expectation of NHS Care: 1 Guidance | Patient Experience in Adult NHS Services: Improving the Experience of Care for People Using Adult NHS Services | Guidance | NICE. https://www.nice.org.uk/guidance/cg138/chapter/Recommendations

Palmer, B., & Rolewicz, L. (2022, September 30). *Peak leaving ? A spotlight on nurse leaver rates in the UK.* Https://Www.Nuffieldtrust.Org.Uk. https://www.nuffieldtrust.org.uk/resource/peak-leaving-a-spotlight-on-nurse-leaver-rates-in-the-uk#:~:text=How%20many%20nurses%20are%20leaving,equivalent%20to%20one%20in%20nine.

Patel, S., Pelletier-Bui, A., Smith, S., Roberts, M. B., Kilgannon, H., Trzeciak, S., & Roberts, B. W. (2019). Curricula for empathy and compassion training in medical education: A systematic review. *PLoS ONE, 14*(8), 1–25. https://doi.org/10.1371/journal.pone.0221412

Sinclair, S., McClement, S., Raffin-Bouchal, S., Hack, T. F., Hagen, N. A., McConnell, S., & Chochinov, H. M. (2016). Compassion in health care: An empirical model. *Journal of Pain and Symptom Management, 51*(2), 193–203. https://doi.org/10.1016/j.jpainsymman.2015.10.009

Thienprayoon, R., Sinclair, S., Lown, B. A., Pestian, T., Awtrey, E., Winick, N., & Kanov, J. (2022). Organizational compassion: Ameliorating healthcare worker's suffering and burnout. *Journal of Wellness, 4*(1), 3–5. https://doi.org 10.55504/2578-9333.1122

Trzeciak, S., & Mazzarelli, A. (2019). *Compassionomics* (First edition). Studer Group.

West, M. A. (2021). *Compassionate Leadership*. Swirling Leaf Press.

2 Empathy, empathic concern, compassion and kindness

Compassion is a complex phenomenon and one that continues to elude complete understanding (Goetz et al., 2010; Mascaro, 2024). Nonetheless, it is a quality of care that healthcare workers try to provide and patients seek on a daily basis. This chapter sets out current ways of understanding empathy, empathic concern, compassion and kindness, terms that are sometimes used interchangeably.

Empathy and empathic concern

Empathy is thought to be an essential building block of compassion but does not necessarily imply care or concern alone. So, for example, just as it is possible to intuitively know or to imagine how someone might feel with the intention of finding the best way of relieving their suffering, it is equally possible to imagine how someone might feel in a particular situation and then, on the basis of that knowledge, manipulate or exploit them for personal gain (Ricard, 2015c).

Notably, empathy can also be complex in healthcare settings where it may arise from a variety of other general or quite specific motivations that may not always be conducive to good care (Batson, 2017; Gilbert, 2020). For example, being sensitive to and motivated to be of benefit to those who have a physical illness, but less so to people whose suffering originates from within a distressed or disturbed state of mind (Gilbert, 2020), can be problematic for both patients and staff. Some empathic responses that spontaneously arise can be unhealthy for the healthcare workforce because they cause distress and depletion in the face of continual exposure to suffering (Ekman & Ekman, 2017; McGonigal, 2022; Schwan, 2018). Repeated experiences of distress caused by some empathic states can also lead to burnout in healthcare workers due to an overidentification with the ongoing suffering (McGonigal, 2022), where the healthcare worker becomes overly fused with, and incapacitated by, the experience of the distress shared with the patient.

DOI: 10.4324/9781003427247-2

Empathic concern is thought to be a motivational state that drives an altruistic response with the aim of relieving suffering in another person, regardless of the perceived cause of the suffering (Batson, 2017). That is, empathic concern for another person is thought necessary for a truly compassionate response.

Empathising with another person's suffering, however, necessarily involves some activation of the same specialised neural networks that are activated in the first-person experience of that misfortune (Singer & Klimecki, 2014), so there is some involuntary and unavoidable 'sharing' of the unpleasant emotional tone of the suffering experience. This process represents a degree of activation of the threat processing system and consequently, attention becomes self-focused rather than turned towards addressing the needs of the person who is suffering. This reactivity of the threat processing system is also associated with behaviours that may further impede a compassionate response, for example, withdrawing from the patient in order to manage one's own distress or to escape the situation (Singer & Klimecki, 2014). Empathising with another's suffering, however, is a necessary part of a compassionate response because it involves the recognition or identification of ongoing suffering and the possibility of offering compassion to relieve that same suffering.

Empathy, or empathic concern, in the context of healthcare requires that the sense of an effective, professional self remains intact and there is only brief, if any fusion with the suffering of the patient in order to respond with appropriate and skilled care and with compassion. Empathy training in the healthcare professions is not unusual, but often varies in methodology and outcomes (e.g., Patel et al., 2019; Riess et al., 2012; Samarasekera et al., 2023), and there is often no distinction made between empathy and compassion. Typically, however, all empathy or compassion trainings in healthcare emphasise the importance of attuning to the ongoing emotional state of oneself as well as to the emotional state of the patient in order to act effectively and with compassion.

Focus Box 2.1   Empathy

Is the same as, or becomes, 'empathic concern' in healthcare because the motivation or intention is to benefit the patient
Helps in the recognition of suffering
Involves unpleasant emotions on exposure to the suffering of another person
Can lead to a withdrawal from the situation as a result of physical sensations, thoughts, and emotions experienced as unpleasant and that are unhelpful in the context
Activates distinct neural circuitry

Compassion

It has been reliably demonstrated that the neural circuitry in the brain activated during an empathic response is different from the neural circuitry that is activated during the compassionate response itself (Bernhardt & Singer, 2012; Engen & Singer, 2013; Singer & Klimecki, 2014). In contrast to empathy, a compassionate response recruits specialised neural circuitry associated with the experience of pleasant emotional feelings (Singer & Klimecki, 2014) and is thought to involve stimulation of the oxytocin-opiate-parasympathetic system (Gilbert, 2020). Activation of this system is also associated with a shift away from the safety seeking preoccupations of oneself triggered by the threat processing system in an empathic response, towards attending to the suffering of another person and a consequent increased likelihood of compassionate action.

Definitions of compassion

Following a review of definitions of compassion, Strauss and colleagues devised a multi-component definition of compassion consisting of

> the recognition of suffering, understanding the universality of suffering in human experience, feeling sympathy, empathy or concern for the person suffering (emotional resonance), tolerating distress associated with witnessing the suffering and the motivation to act or acting to alleviate the suffering.
>
> (Strauss et al., 2016, p. 25)

Other definitions for compassion in healthcare specifically, often derived from qualitative research with patients, have also been proposed and emphasise the relational nature of the action required to relieve suffering. For example, 'the recognition, empathic understanding of and emotional resonance with concerns, pain, distress or suffering of others coupled with motivation and relational actions to ameliorate these conditions' (Lown & MacIntosh, 2014, p. 5). Similarly, 'a virtuous response that seeks to address the suffering and needs of a person through relational understanding and action' (Sinclair et al., 2016, p. 195). Halifax, however, in addition to the relational dimension of compassion that is implicit in her work, emphasises the 'contingent and emergent' nature of compassion (Halifax, 2012, p. 228).

Compassion can also usefully be thought of as including the prevention of suffering in another person (Gilbert, 2019), and different tones of compassion have also been described. Compassion can refer to a tender nurturance (Jazaieri et al., 2013, 2014), a fierce compassion (Neff, 2023) or a compassion that is fuelled by courage (Gilbert, 2021). Furthermore, compassion is known to be both a 'trait' quality, that is, an enduring characteristic, and a 'state' quality, one that may be increased on a temporary basis (Goetz et al., 2010) but also an increased quality of heart that changes from state to trait over time in response to training (Ricard, 2015a).

Three flows of compassion

Gilbert suggests that it is helpful to understand that there are three flows of compassion (2009). Firstly, there is the flow of compassion to oneself (self-compassion), and in this case one is both the individual offering compassion and the recipient of one's own offering of compassion. Secondly, there is the flow of compassion from oneself towards others, and thirdly, the flow of compassion offered to oneself from other people. He also suggests that in order to be able to 'use' compassion, both for oneself and for others, it is important to have experienced compassion as a recipient in primary care giving relationships (Gilbert, 2020).

Self-compassion has been further elaborated on and is described as compassion directed towards oneself in the context of personal suffering, just as one might offer compassion to a friend in trouble (Neff, 2011). Self-compassion as taught in specialist training courses developed by Professors Kristin Neff and Christopher Germer draws on both mindfulness and a sense of common humanity in addition, and self-compassion is proven to be helpful in accepting personal shortcomings and wider challenges faced in the course of one's life (Neff, 2023).

Focus box 2.2   Compassion

Is associated with pleasant emotions
Is associated with approaching the person who is suffering to help them
Activates specialised neural circuitry that is distinct from that activated in an empathic response
Is different from empathic concern

Empathy or compassion fatigue

There are some differences of opinion about these two terms and, as a result, how they are used. McGonigal (2022) describes compassion fatigue in the context of healthcare as being a state of psychological depletion that occurs when there are repeated experiences of system failures or situational factors that prevent or otherwise block a compassionate response.

Therefore, from this point of view, it is possible that compassion fatigue can be seen as a form of, or a contributing factor to, moral injury in healthcare workers, characterised as a state of psychological distress resulting from acts of omission or commission that transgress the moral or ethical code of the individual involved (Litz et al., 2009). Ricard (2015b) prefers the term empathy fatigue in association with burnout. This is on the basis of the understanding that compassion is associated with positive emotions and does not become weary or wear out those who experience it.

In this text, the term empathy fatigue is preferred, although in combination with McGonigal's description of the causation of compassion fatigue. This is because in health and social care practice, it often appears to be the case that workers report being prevented from moving from a state of empathic concern that necessarily involves unpleasant emotions, to the enactment of compassion and consequent feelings of personal and professional satisfaction because of the constraints of the systems that they work in.

Oxytocin, vasopressin and compassion

The neuropeptides oxytocin and vasopressin have long been linked to the nuance of friendly and cooperative behaviours in humans, including those of compassionate care giving relationships (MacDonald & MacDonald, 2010). Furthermore, the way that the two neuropeptides work in individuals is thought to be influenced by early experiences of receiving care and compassion. Oxytocin as part of the oxytocin-opiate-parasympathetic system active in compassion appears to play a part in reducing unpleasant emotional arousal or feelings on exposure to suffering, whilst vasopressin appears to be associated with rapid, defensive mobilisation and threat vigilance in response to stressful experiences (Carter et al., 2017).

Kindness

Kindness is often grouped with compassion as part of a 'family' of words in describing a desirable quality of care (e.g., National Institute for Health and Social Care Excellence, 2021). Unsurprisingly, the practice of kindness is strongly implicated in healthy team functioning and thought to reduce errors in healthcare (Fryburg, 2023). Being kind to others is known to have some modest benefit for oneself no matter who the recipient is (Curry et al., 2018), and this effect also extends to a positive benefit that is obtained when other people witness an act of kindness (Rowland & Curry, 2019). In an exploration of kindness within healthcare specifically, Hake and Post (2023) tentatively define kindness as a simple action, immediately perceived by the recipient as a positive experience. The same authors suggest that kindness may be more easily taught in a medical curriculum than compassion and would provide a starting point for later teaching on the more complex nature of compassion. Possible objections to this, however, would include the view that the discretionary nature of kindness, without any accompanying professional or ethical sensitivity, may simply become a form of favouritism and perpetuate and worsen existing inequities in healthcare settings (Jesudason, 2023). Furthermore, most definitions of compassion agree that it is 'suffering-specific' (Strauss et al., 2016), and whilst kindness is important in healthcare, it is insufficient to address suffering because compassion in healthcare often requires a range of specialist and professional skills developed to relieve suffering.

Summary points

Empathic concern is a necessary pre-cursor to compassion

It is important to consider the negative experience of empathic concern on healthcare workers and how to best deal with it

Compassion can be expressed in different 'tones'

Compassion can be expressed towards oneself or other people, or experienced as being offered from other people.

Oxytocin and vasopressin have different roles in empathy and compassion but both are involved

Compassion is regarded as suffering-specific, unlike kindness

References

Batson, C. D. (2017). The empathy-altruism hypothesis: What and so what? In E. M. Seppala, E. Simon-Thomas, S. L. Brown, M. C. Worline, D. C. Cameron, & J. R. Doty (Eds.), *The Oxford Handbook of Compassion Science* (First edition, pp. 27–40). Oxford University Press.

Bernhardt, B. C., & Singer, T. (2012). The neural basis of empathy. In *Annual Review of Neuroscience* (Vol. 35, pp. 1–23). https://doi.org/10.1146/annurev-neuro-062111-150536

Carter, C. S., Ben-Ami Bartal, I., & Porges, E. C. (2017). The roots of compassion: An evolutionary and neurobiological perspective. In E. M. Seppala, E. Simon-Thomas, S. L. Brown, M. C. Worline, C. D. Cameron, & J. R. Doty (Eds.), *The Oxford Book of Compassion Science* (First edition, pp. 173–187). Oxford University Press.

Curry, O. S., Rowland, L. A., Van Lissa, C. J., Zlotowitz, S., McAlaney, J., & Whitehouse, H. (2018). Happy to help? A systematic review and meta-analysis of the effects of performing acts of kindness on the well-being of the actor. *Journal of Experimental Social Psychology*, *76*, 320–329. https://doi.org/10.1016/j.jesp.2018.02.014

Ekman, P., & Ekman, E. (2017). Is global compassion achievable? In E. M. Seppala, E. Simon-Thomas, S. L. Brown, M. C. Worline, D. C. Cameron, & J. R. Doty (Eds.), *The Oxford Handbook of Compassion Science* (First edition, pp. 41–49). Oxford University Press.

Engen, H. G., & Singer, T. (2013). Empathy circuits. In *Current Opinion in Neurobiology*. https://doi.org/10.1016/j.conb.2012.11.003

Fryburg, D. A. (2023). Kindness isn't just about being nice: The value proposition of kindness as viewed through the lens of incivility in the healthcare workplace. *Behavioral Sciences*, *13*(6), 457. https://doi.org/10.3390/bs13060457

Gilbert, P. (2009). Expressing the compassionate mind. In *The Compassionate Mind: A New Approach to Life's Challenges* (First edition, pp. 416–446). New Harbinger Publications Inc.

Gilbert, P. (2019). Explorations into the nature and function of compassion. *Current Opinion in Psychology*, *28*, 108–114. https://doi.org/https://doi.org/10.1016/j.copsyc.2018.12.002

Gilbert, P. (2020). Compassion: From its evolution to a psychotherapy. *Frontiers in Psychology*, *11*(December). https://doi.org/10.3389/fpsyg.2020.586161

Gilbert, P. (2021). Creating a compassionate world: Addressing the conflicts between sharing and caring versus controlling and holding evolved strategies. *Frontiers in Psychology*, *11*(February). https://doi.org/10.3389/fpsyg.2020.582090

Goetz, J. L., Keltner, D., & Simon-Thomas, E. (2010). Compassion: An evolutionary analysis and empirical review. *Psychological Bulletin*, *136*(3), 351–374. https://doi.org/10.1037/a0018807

Hake, A. B., & Post, S. G. (2023). Kindness: Definitions and a pilot study for the development of a kindness scale in healthcare. *PloS One*, *18*(7), e0288766. https://doi.org/10.1371/journal.pone.0288766

Halifax, J. (2012). A heuristic model of enactive compassion. In *Current Opinion in Supportive and Palliative Care* (Vol. 6, Issue 2, pp. 228–235). https://doi.org/10.1097/SPC.0b013e3283530fbe

Jazaieri, H., Jinpa, G. T., McGonigal, K., Rosenberg, E. L., Finkelstein, J., Simon-Thomas, E., Cullen, M., Doty, J. R., Gross, J. J., & Goldin, P. R. (2013). Enhancing compassion: A randomized controlled trial of a compassion cultivation training program. *Journal of Happiness Studies*, *14*(4), 1113–1126. https://doi.org/10.1007/s10902-012-9373-z

Jazaieri, H., McGonigal, K., Jinpa, T., Doty, J. R., Gross, J. J., & Goldin, P. R. (2014). A randomized controlled trial of compassion cultivation training: Effects on mindfulness, affect, and emotion regulation. *Motivation and Emotion*, *38*(1), 23–35. https://doi.org/10.1007/s11031-013-9368-z

Jesudason, E. (2023). Ethical problems with kindness in healthcare. *Journal of Medical Ethics*, *49*, 558–562. doi:10.1136/medethics-2022-108357

Litz, B. T., Stein, N., Delaney, E., Lebowitz, L., Nash, W. P., Silva, C., & Maguen, S. (2009). Moral injury and moral repair in war veterans: A preliminary model and intervention strategy. In *Clinical Psychology Review* (Vol. 29, Issue 8, pp. 695–706). https://doi.org/10.1016/j.cpr.2009.07.003

Lown, B., & MacIntosh, S. (2014). *Recommendations from a Conference on Advancing Compassionate, Person-and Family-Centered Care Through Interprofessional Education for Collaborative Practice.* https://www.theschwartzcenter.org/media/FINAL-Triple-C-Conference-Recommendations-Report.pdf

MacDonald, K., & MacDonald, T. M. (2010). The peptide that binds: A systematic review of Oxytocin and its prosocial effects in humans. In *Harvard Review of Psychiatry* (Vol. 18, Issue 1, pp. 1–21). https://doi.org/10.3109/10673220903523615

Mascaro, J. (2024, August). *The Science of Compassion.* Mind and Life Institute. https://www.mindandlife.org/insight/the-science-of-compassion/

McGonigal, K. (2022, April 20). The practical science of compassion. *Compassion in Therapy Summit. Free Online Event. Hosted by the Awake Network.*

National Institute for Health and Social Care Excellence. (2021, June 21). *Clinical Guideline 138. Patient experience in adult NHS services: Improving the experience of care for people using adult NHS services for the patient.* NICE Guideline 138 Experience Which Outlines the General Expectation of NHS Care: 1 Guidance | Patient Experience in Adult NHS Services: Improving the Experience of Care for People Using Adult NHS Services | Guidance | NICE. https://www.nice.org.uk/guidance/cg138/chapter/1-Guidance#knowing-the-patient-as-an-individual

Neff, K. D. (2011). Self-compassion, self-esteem, and well-being. *Social and Personality Psychology Compass, 5*(1), 1–12. https://doi.org/10.1111/j.1751-9004.2010.00330.x

Neff, K. D. (2023). Self-compassion: Theory, method, research, and intervention. *Annual Review of Psychology, 74*, 193–218.

Patel, S., Pelletier-Bui, A., Smith, S., Roberts, M. B., Kilgannon, H., Trzeciak, S., & Roberts, B. W. (2019). Curricula for empathy and compassion training in medical education: A systematic review. *PLoS ONE, 14*(8), 1–25. https://doi.org/10.1371/journal.pone.0221412

Ricard, M. (2015a). Can we change? In *Altruism. The power of compassion to change yourself and the world* (First edition, pp. 239–246). Little, Brown and Company.

Ricard, M. (2015b). From empathy to compassion in a Neuroscience Laboratory. In *Altruism. The power of compassion to change yourself and the world* (pp. 56–64). Little, Brown and Company.

Ricard, M. (2015c). What is empathy? In *Altruism. The power of compassion to change yourself and the world: Vol. First edition* (pp. 39–55). Little, Brown and Company.

Riess, H., Kelley, J. M., Bailey, R. W., Dunn, E. J., & Phillips, M. (2012). Empathy training for resident physicians: A randomized controlled trial of a neuroscience-informed curriculum. *Journal of General Internal Medicine, 27*(10), 1280–1286. https://doi.org/10.1007/s11606-012-2063-z

Rowland, L., & Curry, O. S. (2019). A range of kindness activities boost happiness. In *Journal of Social Psychology* (Vol. 159, Issue 3, pp. 340–343). Routledge. https://doi.org/10.1080/00224545.2018.1469461

Samarasekera, D. D., Lee, S. S., Yeo, J. H. T., Yeo, S. P., & Ponnamperuma, G. (2023). Empathy in health professions education: What works, gaps and areas for improvement. *Medical Education, 57*(1), 86–101. https://doi.org/10.1111/medu.14865

Schwan, D. (2018). Should physicians be empathetic? Rethinking clinical empathy. *Theoretical Medicine and Bioethics, 39*(5), 347–360. https://doi.org/10.1007/s11017-018-9463-y

Sinclair, S., McClement, S., Raffin-Bouchal, S., Hack, T. F., Hagen, N. A., McConnell, S., & Chochinov, H. M. (2016). Compassion in health care: An empirical model. *Journal of Pain and Symptom Management, 51*(2), 193–203. https://doi.org/10.1016/j.jpainsymman.2015.10.009

Singer, T., & Klimecki, O. M. (2014). Empathy and compassion. In *Current Biology* (Vol. 24, Issue 18, pp. R875–R878). https://doi.org/10.1016/j.cub.2014.06.054

Strauss, C., Lever Taylor, B., Gu, J., Kuyken, W., Baer, R., Jones, F., & Cavanagh, K. (2016). What is compassion and how can we measure it? A review of definitions and measures. *Clinical Psychology Review, 47*, 15–27. https://doi.org/10.1016/j.cpr.2016.05.004

3 Compassion

Embodied and evolved

This chapter draws on the body of work by Professor Paul Gilbert, who has demonstrated that compassion is best understood as an evolved psychosocial process. The chapter focuses on the embodied nature of threat and safety and the co-creation of safe relationships through behavioural vectors as the basis for compassion. Furthermore, the chapter references the health implications of states of threat and calm and describes how personal experiences shape perceptions of safety.

The capacity to be compassionate is a shared evolutionary heritage for all human beings and evolved as an integral part of the mammalian care giving system that was a critical factor in ensuring survival and reproduction in early human societies (Goetz et al., 2010). The compassion and care giving system was integral to the formation of family groups, as well as an increasing number of relationships with others for a variety of needs, as societal connections between people developed in number and complexity (Gilbert, 2020). Understanding the human need to feel safe as a pre-cursor to the expression and experience of compassion is important in understanding the nature of compassion in contemporary healthcare settings. Key to the human experience of safety is the functioning of the autonomic nervous system (ANS).

The autonomic nervous system

In humans, the ANS is responsible for connecting internal organs to the brain and for regulating unconscious processes such as body temperature and breathing. The two branches of the ANS are the sympathetic nervous system (SNS) and the parasympathetic nervous system (PNS). The SNS is a major component of the threat processing system; it operates on the 'smoke detector principle' where it is inactive for much of the time when conditions are safe but is rapidly activated if danger or threat are identified. The PNS is responsible, along with other supporting bodily systems, for calming and soothing when there is safety.

DOI: 10.4324/9781003427247-3

Behavioural responses to threat

There are three ways that humans respond, depending upon the level of threat severity (Porges, 1997). The most extreme behavioural response of all is a 'freeze' or faint response that is elicited in situations that represent a very high level of threat. Animals may become immobile and appear lifeless when subject to predation with little chance of escape. This is a temporary immobilisation that is reversible once the danger recedes and there is an opportunity for escape. Humans share a version of this dramatic response with animals if actual or perceived danger is extreme, for example, in conflict situations or sometimes in threatening social situations where people find themselves 'freezing' with fear.

If the degree of threat is less severe, but present nonetheless, strong activation of the SNS provokes a 'fight or flight' response in order to either confront and overcome or escape from the source of danger. A third response to somewhat lower levels of interpersonal threat involves using evolutionarily newer capacities of mind such as thinking and reasoning about how to engage another person to reduce the threat level, rather than to flee, submit to them or fight them. This involves engaging the other person with words and non-verbal behaviour that help to co-create feelings of safety and encouragement and so suppresses activation of the threat processing system. The co-creation of feelings of safety and mutuality also describes a process of emotional co-regulation, whereby the fluctuating emotions of two people, through talking and non-verbal behaviour, come to resonate with each other (Butler & Randall, 2013).

If these newer adaptations of the nervous system concerned with forming relationships with other people to co-create safety and cooperation do not provide safety, the next configuration of primitive neural circuitry down is activated, along with the accompanying behaviour typical for that response (Porges, 1997). So, for example, if talking and reasoning does not calm someone down, or if the source of threat remains high or even increases, the flight or fight response will be triggered. If the threat of harm remains extreme and neither escape nor confrontation appear to offer the possibility of safety, then the freeze state may be triggered as a response of last resort.

Focus box 3.1   Three ways of responding to threat

Freeze
Fight/flight or submissive behaviour (backing down)
Engaging with someone who presents a threat to co-create feelings of safety and build a mutually beneficial relationship (emotional co-regulation)

Safety and safeness

Professor Gilbert has drawn on a number of scientific disciplines and theories, including that of attachment theory, over several decades to produce a large body of scholarly work on compassion (e.g., Gilbert, 2015, 2019, 2020, 2021). He has demonstrated the importance and distinction between states of safety and safeness that have their roots in two opposing neurophysiological systems. These are sensitive systems shaped by childhood experience that can either help or hinder the capacity to express or experience compassion in adult life (Gilbert, 2020).

The threat processing system is thought to include the SNS and involvement of the amygdala and pituitary-adrenal axis. The threat processing system becomes activated in the presence of danger or threat but 'steps down', although remains vigilant (as in the smoke detector principle) in the absence of threat. Feelings of anxiety and fear and self-focused, safety seeking behaviours are also associated with activation of the threat processing system. *Safety* is defined as the absence of threat and relates specifically to the threat processing system. Feelings of *safeness*, and accompanying feelings of calm and encouragement, however are of a different nature because they are thought to originate from active stimulation of the oxytocin-opiate PNS circuitry. Stimulation of this system is capable of deactivating or suppressing threat processing even when some degree of threat is present (Gilbert, 2020). Furthermore, when there is no ongoing threat processing, other more varied and creative mind states can emerge because there is no preoccupation with safety seeking and care and attention can be deployed freely.

When the body and mind are in this more easeful state, metabolic resources are also available to repair routine 'wear and tear' in the body incurred in the course of daily life. This is in contrast to the absorption of metabolic resources in preparation for defensive action or the defensive action itself when the threat processing system is activated, (Porges, 1997, 2017, 2022).

A cascade of other physiological effects, for example changes in the immune system, are also associated with activation of the threat processing system and are known to have negative effects on psychological and physical health in the long term if periods of threat reactivity are prolonged (Thayer et al., 2010). Importantly, in order for compassion to be both expressed and experienced, it is necessary for the threat processing system to be sufficiently suppressed to allow stimulation of the oxytocin-opiate-parasympathetic circuitry. Feelings of safeness are then able to emerge and form the basis and context for a compassionate interaction (Gilbert, 2020).

Focus box 3.2   Two different evolved and embodied systems

The threat processing system consisting of the amygdala, pituitary-
adrenal axis and the sympathetic nervous system
Safety is experienced when there is no or minimal activation of the
threat processing system
The calm-caring-compassion system consisting of oxytocin-opiate-
parasympathetic nervous system circuitry
Safeness is experienced when the compassion system is actively
stimulated

Communication and emotional co-regulation

The underlying mechanisms and pathways responsible for linking human
communication, emotional co-regulation and compassion are complex
and incompletely understood. The existence of some form of emotionally co-regulating system in humans, as an integral part of compassion,
however, is not in doubt (Gilbert, 2019; Halifax, 2012; Siegel, 2019) and
patients often report a visceral experience of connectedness in response
to what they name as compassion (e.g., Sinclair et al., 2016). Calming and soothing patients who are unwell or distressed, by talking to
them and sometimes using touch, is also a daily experience for many
healthcare workers. In a systematic review of training courses for doctors, increasing awareness of their own bodily position and proximity in
relation to the patient, careful use of speech and eye gaze and attention
to the emotional state of the patient were all behaviours consistently
associated with improvements in the expression of compassion or empathy, although the authors noted that not all studies included in the review
evaluated the experience of compassion from a patient perspective (Patel
et al., 2019).

Whilst much has been written about the Polyvagal Theory and the
Social Engagement System in relation to both safety and compassion
(Porges, 1997, 2009, 2017), more recently, the theories have become the
focus of some criticism (Grossman, 2023). The same behavioural vectors
involved in conveying compassion as described by Porges, however, are
the same as those identified in the study above by Patel and colleagues
(2019). Porges theorises that humans are thought to convey the degree
of either SNS reactivity related to threat processing or the degree of
PNS-mediated influence, indicating a state more conducive to safety and

cooperation, through and with their facial expression, tone of voice and patterns of bodily movement. Porges goes on to say that without any conscious awareness, these bio-behavioural signals are rapidly 'de-coded' as either those that offer the likelihood of a safe social encounter, or those communicating high levels of SNS unstable reactivity and the need to be wary and to remain distant.

Porges (1997, 2009) also proposes that interactions with another person consist of a moment-by-moment, two-way stream of powerful bio-behavioural signals. This flow of changing signals is reflective of underlying shifts in neurophysiology relating to states of threat and safety, of all magnitudes, with behavioural vectors 'livestreaming' the possibilities, or lack thereof, of safe engagement. Furthermore, these signals are, by design, mutually influencing, and it is possible, either knowingly or unknowingly, to influence the ANS of another person with one's own bio-behavioural signals, and so to emotionally co-regulate someone to a state of fearful SNS reactivity and threat processing, or to stimulate PNS influence to calm and soothe. Intentionally transmitting bio-behavioural signals of calm steadiness to downregulate or deactivate threat processing in another person so that they feel comforted and soothed is engaging in a process of emotional co-regulation, a form of skilled compassionate action.

Individual differences in sensitivity to threat and safety

Via the process of neuroplasticity (Dan, 2019), the ANS is 'tuned' by experiences of relationships with other people, particularly those of care givers in infancy and childhood (Gilbert, 2009). Repeated experiences of relationships characterised by a lack of safety, neglect and unpredictability mean that threat processing is easily triggered (Gilbert, 2009, 2020; Porges, 2022). Interpersonal strategies involving defence or withdrawal from perceived or actual threat, including those of an existential or social nature, may become overly developed and easily activated. Attunement and responsiveness to the bio-behavioural signals of safety and encouragement to engage from others may also be adversely impacted because of a failure of the PNS and oxytocin-opiate systems to support states of calm that allow such engagement (Gilbert, 2020).

In contrast, repeated and ongoing experiences of relationships characterised by safety and feelings of connectedness result in the ability to engage in healthy relationships as adults (Gilbert, 2009, 2020). When infants and young children are distressed but able to reliably depend upon trusted others to help co-regulate their emotions through the bio-behavioural signals of safety and care conveyed by facial expression, tone of voice and, in particular, touch, there is healthy mental and physical development (Gilbert, 2020). As children grow, they 'internalise' this process of emotional co-regulation by another adult, and the foundation for their own capacity to engage in effective emotional self-regulation is established (Gilbert, 2014). This same foundation also enables a potential for the healthy emotional co-regulation of other people in adult life. Provided that there is sufficient safety (absence of threat, or any threat present is outweighed by signals of safeness), it is possible to be alert and attentive to the needs of others, help to emotionally co-regulate them when in need and so provide care and comfort for another person in turn (Gilbert, 2020).

Because life experiences shape each individual's sensitivity to threat and safety, what is experienced as sufficiently safe will vary within the population as a whole. This variation also extends to the people who work in health and social care settings and those who are use or who are seen in those same settings. The conditions necessary for sufficient safety for one person might breach a threshold of sufficient safety for another, but it is also the case that some situations would not be experienced as sufficiently safe by anyone, for example being confronted by a stranger in the dark, when alone.

Summary points

The capacity to be compassionate is a shared evolutionary heritage

Safe relationships are co-created by the exchange of powerful bio-behavioural signals communicated through facial expression, quality of voice and other behavioural vectors,

These behavioural vectors are thought to reflect underlying neurophysiological states of calm, or activation of the threat processing system

There is a mutually influencing effect between people when they are communicating that can influence the underlying state of calm or preparedness for threat in either person

Communication is a means of emotional co-regulation between people

Individual differences in sensitivity to bio-behavioural signals of threat or safety and calm can result from life experiences that 'tune' the nervous system

Feeling sufficiently safe is a necessary condition for both the experience and expression of compassion

References

Butler, E. A., & Randall, A. K. (2013). Emotional coregulation in close relationships. *Emotion Review, 5*(2), 202–210. https://doi.org/10.1177/1754073912451630

Dan, B. (2019). Neuroscience underlying rehabilitation: What is neuroplasticity? In *Developmental Medicine and Child Neurology* (Vol. 61, Issue 11, p. 1240). Blackwell Publishing Ltd. https://doi.org/10.1111/dmcn.14341

Gilbert, P. (2009). The challenges of life. In *The Compassionate Mind: A New Approach to Life's Challenges* (pp. 21–78). New Harbinger Publications, Inc.

Gilbert, P. (2014). The origins and nature of compassion focused therapy. *British Journal of Clinical Psychology, 53*(1), 6–41. https://doi.org/10.1111/bjc.12043

Gilbert, P. (2015). The evolution and social dynamics of compassion. *Social and Personality Psychology Compass, 9*(6), 239–254. https://doi.org/10.1111/spc3.12176

Gilbert, P. (2019). Explorations into the nature and function of compassion. *Current Opinion in Psychology, 28*, 108–114. https://doi.org/https://doi.org/10.1016/j.copsyc.2018.12.002

Gilbert, P. (2020). Compassion: From its evolution to a psychotherapy. *Frontiers in Psychology, 11*(December). https://doi.org/10.3389/fpsyg.2020.586161

Gilbert, P. (2021). Creating a compassionate world: Addressing the conflicts between sharing and caring versus controlling and holding evolved strategies. *Frontiers in Psychology, 11*(February). https://doi.org/10.3389/fpsyg.2020.582090

Goetz, J. L., Keltner, D., & Simon-Thomas, E. (2010). Compassion: An evolutionary analysis and empirical eeview. *Psychological Bulletin, 136*(3), 351–374. https://doi.org/10.1037/a0018807

Grossman, P. (2023). Fundamental challenges and likely refutations of the five basic premises of the polyvagal theory. In *Biological Psychology* (Vol. 180). Elsevier B.V. https://doi.org/10.1016/j.biopsycho.2023.108589

Halifax, J. (2012). A heuristic model of enactive compassion. In *Current Opinion in Supportive and Palliative Care* (Vol. 6, Issue 2, pp. 228–235). https://doi.org/10.1097/SPC.0b013e3283530fbe

Patel, S., Pelletier-Bui, A., Smith, S., Roberts, M. B., Kilgannon, H., Trzeciak, S., & Roberts, B. W. (2019). Curricula for empathy and compassion training in medical education: A systematic review. *PLoS ONE, 14*(8), 1–25. https://doi.org/10.1371/journal.pone.0221412

Porges, S. W. (1997). Emotion: An evolutionary by-product of the neural regulation of the autonomic nervous system. *Annals of the New York Academy of Sciences, 807*(1), 62–77.

Porges, S. W. (2009). The polyvagal theory: New insights into adaptive reactions of the autonomic nervous system. *Cleveland Clinic Journal of Medicine, 76*(SUPPL.2). https://doi.org/10.3949/ccjm.76.s2.17

Porges, S. W. (2017). Vagal pathways: Portals to compassion. In E. M. Seppala, E. Simon-Thomas, S. L. Brown, M. C. Worline, C. D. Cameron, & J. R. Doty (Eds.), *The Oxford Handbook of Compassion Science* (pp. 189–202). Oxford University Press.

Porges, S. W. (2022). Polyvagal theory: A science of safety. In *Frontiers in Integrative Neuroscience* (Vol. 16). Frontiers Media S.A. https://doi.org/10.3389/fnint.2022.871227

Siegel, D. J. (2019). The mind in psychotherapy: An interpersonal neurobiology framework for understanding and cultivating mental health. *Psychology and Psychotherapy: Theory, Research and Practice, 92*(2), 224–237. https://doi.org/10.1111/papt.12228

Sinclair, S., McClement, S., Raffin-Bouchal, S., Hack, T. F., Hagen, N. A., McConnell, S., & Chochinov, H. M. (2016). Compassion in health care: An empirical model. *Journal of Pain and Symptom Management, 51*(2), 193–203. https://doi.org/10.1016/j.jpainsymman.2015.10.009

Thayer, J. F., Yamamoto, S. S., & Brosschot, J. F. (2010). The relationship of autonomic imbalance, heart rate variability and cardiovascular disease risk factors. In *International Journal of Cardiology* (Vol. 141, Issue 2, pp. 122–131). https://doi.org/10.1016/j.ijcard.2009.09.543

4 The function of compassion in healthcare

This chapter describes the function of compassion as essentially one of emotional co-regulation to preserve safety and dignity for those who are suffering and applies it to contemporary healthcare settings. The implications of this emotional co-regulatory role for healthcare professionals in the context of over-burdened healthcare systems are considered.

There are many different forms of compassion, for example, the compassion shown by people who donate a kidney to strangers in need, or those who rescue abandoned animals. Compassion in healthcare, however, has a very particular place and is a powerful adjunct to healing and recovery. Compassionate care helps to reduce post-operative pain and diabetic complications; it enhances the effects of rehabilitation and has other positive effects for patients, both physical and psychological (see Trzeciak & Mazzarelli, 2019a, 2019b for an overview). There is also a growing body of evidence to suggest that positive physical health outcomes are also associated with higher levels of compassion expressed towards oneself (self-compassion) (e.g., Ferrari et al., 2017; Phillips & Hine, 2021), in addition to positive mental health outcomes. It is proposed that compassionate care contributes to better outcomes through relationships with healthcare professionals that promote a healthy neurophysiological state supportive of healing and restoration. A compassionate and supportive relationship with oneself, as opposed to a harsh and critical relationship with oneself is thought to work in the same way.

The respectful and emotional co-regulatory function of compassion

Porges (2017) describes the evolutionary function of compassion as allowing those who are sick or suffering to be seen to be vulnerable without feeling shameful or fearful of being attacked in some way. He proposes that the negative feelings triggered on exposure to the suffering of other people (and that necessarily form part of an empathic response) reduces the likelihood that the sufferer will be shamed by the

DOI: 10.4324/9781003427247-4

onlooker because in that brief moment, the onlooker is also sharing in those unpleasant feelings of pain and vulnerability. He goes on to say that compassion is an inherently respectful process 'and contributes to the healing process by empowering the other' (Porges, 2017, p. 90).

Porges's description of the function of compassion is particularly pertinent to the work of healthcare professionals because healthcare-related shame is very commonly reported by patients (e.g., Dolezal, 2022; Jaeb & Pecanac, 2024). Shame itself has been described as both an isolating emotion (MacDonald & Morley, 2001) and a state of mind based on the idea that other people are potentially rejecting or hostile (Gilbert, 2007) and, as a result, shame acts as a very effective trigger for the threat processing system.

People may also feel shameful about other aspects of their lifestyle that are inadvertently revealed when they come into contact with professionals in healthcare systems, for example, homelessness or food insecurity.

Somewhat obviously, illness, or the need for contact with health or social care services can also provoke feelings of vulnerability and so act as a very effective trigger for the threat processing system. Consequently, a further, and possibly more familiar role for healthcare professionals is the emotional co-regulation of states of health-related fear and anxiety, emotional states that may extend to the people who are close to the patient.

Focus box 4.1   Two main areas of respectful, emotional co-regulation for patients in healthcare

Health-related shame
Health-related fear and anxiety

Respectful, emotional co-regulation competencies

A wide range of health and social care workers are entrusted with promoting respectful and caring relationships with the patients or service users that they have contact with. This includes all patient-facing staff, for example, the healthcare workers who provide housekeeping and hospitality support to inpatient units in hospitals or long-term care in residential facilities and who may be in close contact with vulnerable people (e.g., National Institute for Health and Social Care Excellence, 2021). From this point of view, a respectful and emotional co-regulatory function of compassion has relevance for most, if not all, healthcare staff and especially for those who have a professional clinical training. This application of the function of compassion to healthcare suggests two broad role-related professional competencies for the healthcare professionals in relation to the people in their care.

The first role-related competency is for healthcare workers *to bear professional witness to the suffering and vulnerability of the people that they care for, without triggering feelings of health-related shame or fear.* This first competency is aligned with the need to avoid triggering the threat processing system involving SNS reactivity, the amygdala and the pituitary-adrenal axis (Gilbert, 2014). Avoiding triggering this fearful response allows metabolic resources to be used for healing and restoration (Porges, 2017) in patients, rather than being deployed in the service of a defensive reaction.

The second role-related competency is for healthcare workers to *intentionally use their professional skills, including those of a relational and communicative nature, to alleviate and prevent suffering, including feelings of health-related shame and fear.* Specifically, this competency relates to actively stimulating the oxytocin-opiate-parasympathetic system to offer comfort. This process involves co-creating feelings of safety and encouragement that promote a physiological state conducive to healing and restoration and one that is often experienced as a mutual feeling of connection between healthcare personnel and their patients (e.g., Perry, 2008; Sinclair et al., 2016). Metabolic resources are available to be used for healing and restoration in this state because the activity of the threat processing system has been sufficiently suppressed.

Both the first and second role-related competencies are practised within the bounds of the professional relationship between the healthcare worker and the patient. This is a safe and respectful relationship that is negotiated between the two participants, albeit each with different roles and responsibilities in the encounter. Importantly, the responsibility on the part of the healthcare worker involved is necessarily inclusive of any other profession-specific competencies necessary for the care of the patient (Halifax, 2012, 2013; Heinze et al., 2020).

In practice, the flow of the interaction is likely to be coordinated by the healthcare worker because they possess specialist knowledge and have a particular understanding of the context of the encounter that needs to be shared with the patient. The nature of the relationship, however, is co-created with the quality of the exchange of bio-behavioural signalling through means of facial expression, tone of voice and bodily proximity.

Focus box 4.2   Effect of oxytocin-opiate-parasympathetic influence in patients

Promotes feelings of safety and encouragement
Is supportive of healing and restoration
Can enable feelings of presence and connection with the healthcare worker

Safety and compassion

It is important to understand that feeling safe is the key factor in both the expression of compassion by healthcare professionals and the experience of compassion as it is felt by patients. The expression or experience of compassion is not possible if safety is lacking and the threat processing system has been triggered strongly. The system responsible for threat processing and the system that is involved in co-creating safety and connection for compassion are mutually opposing systems. For the most part, when one is 'online', the opposing system is inhibited, although the threat processing system can be sufficiently 'deactivated' or suppressed by signs of safeness so that the oxytocin-opiate-parasympathetic system can be active and predominate in influence. Because the threat processing system is part of the autonomic nervous system, it continues to operate in the background and is able to be activated rapidly in response to any increase in threat level, if required.

The conditions necessary for patients to experience compassion

Feeling safe for patients means that any source of threat present is outweighed by the value of other cues of safeness that are also present at the same time. This means that the cues of safeness transmitted by the healthcare worker through facial expression, gaze, words and tone of voice are sufficient to disable or inhibit strong threat processing system activation. Alternatively, the patient is receptive to stimulation of the oxytocin-opiate-parasympathetic system via those same behavioural vectors. As a result, the patient is able to feel calm, and encouraged by the healthcare worker within the encounter, even in the face of some degree of threat.

For example, receiving a serious diagnosis or being informed about the prospect of significant surgery would represent a serious threat for most people. It is easy to see how either of these events would trigger the threat processing system and provoke associated feelings of anxiety, or even anger. The involvement in the clinic, however, of a competent healthcare professional who is a skilled communicator and in whom the patient has confidence can act as a potent cue of safeness to reduce the sense of ongoing threat. This then helps the patient to feel supported and encouraged and increases the likelihood that the encounter will be experienced as a compassionate connection, both in the moment and in an 'internalised' way at a later date when it is recalled to mind (Gilbert, 2020).

Emotion co-regulation and the workforce

Compassion is regarded as an essential quality of good leadership in health and social care for important reasons, including for the well-being of the workforce (see West, 2021, for a comprehensive overview). Members of the healthcare workforce, for the most part, are not vulnerable to health-related shame and fear in the same way as patients, at least at work although, at times, some people undoubtedly have crises or find themselves in situations that leave them in need of compassion from work colleagues.

It is the case, though, that currently, many healthcare workers feel over-burdened with work responsibilities and are angry or anxious about their working conditions (e.g., Thienprayoon et al., 2022), and these feelings in themselves are consistent with some activation of the threat processing system. Consequently, dependent upon the degree of activation and the degree of support (or signals of safeness) available to offset this sense of threat, it can make it difficult for healthcare professionals to offer compassion to the people in their care.

The function of compassion in relation to the workforce differs from the function in relation to patients but has some relevance and could still be usefully considered and applied in the following way: The first objective then is for all levels of healthcare workers *to avoid triggering feelings of fear in their co-workers or of causing them to feel demeaned.* This objective is aligned with the need to avoid triggering the threat processing system involving SNS reactivity, the amygdala and the pituitary-adrenal axis. When there is activation of the threat processing system, there are typically feelings of fear or anger, and attention becomes focused on the self rather than on other people, and thinking becomes contracted around seeking safety and loses flexibility. Avoiding triggering a fearful response allows metabolic resources to be used for the restoration of routine bodily 'wear and tear' rather than being deployed in the service of a defensive reaction (Porges, 2017) or contributing to other unwanted physiological effects, known to be associated with poor health outcomes in the long-term (Thayer et al., 2010).

The second objective is for healthcare workers to *act together in a professional manner to intentionally promote safe, collegial and respectful working.* This second objective speaks to a collective responsibility for the co-creation of safe relationships between members of the workforce. When relationships are conducted in ways that actively stimulate the oxytocin-opiate-parasympathetic system, feelings of safety and connection are reinforced and promoted between members of the workforce. The activation of the same system can also help to reduce excessive rivalry or competitive behaviour (Gilbert, 2020) that is sometimes seen within healthcare systems and relationships conducted in this way also promote a healthy physiological state that is supportive of mental and physical well-being.

Furthermore, compassion is just one of a number of other qualities of mind that can emerge when people feel sufficiently safe and when the

Table 4.1 Comparison of effects on healthcare personnel of activation of the threat processing system compared with oxytocin-opiate parasympathetic nervous system stimulation

Oxytocin-opiate-parasympathetic influence	Threat processing system activated
Feelings of satisfaction, creativity and community	Feelings of fear, anxiety and anger
Enables an outward focus on others and productive engagement with work	Narrow focus on the self and safety-seeking behaviour
Enables effective expression of compassion to patients	Incompatible with effective expression of compassion
Promotes health and well-being in the short term and long term	Long-term threat processing system activation associated with poor long-term health outcomes

oxytocin-opiate-parasympathetic system is stimulated. More expansive states of mind that are conducive to creative and innovative thinking and ways of working can develop and are key features of a workforce aligned to provide compassionate care to others see table 4.1. West (2021) suggests that the role of leadership in health and social care is to both embody compassion and to cultivate the conditions that are conducive to compassionate care.

Conditions of safety for healthcare workers

For healthcare workers, feeling safe (or sufficiently safe) means that any cues of safeness that are present outweigh or compensate for any threat present, so it may not be necessary to eliminate all sources of threat in order to feel safe.

For example, a behaviourally disturbed patient in the ER, would present a clear threat likely to trigger the threat processing system in many people. In the presence of cues of safeness, however, namely adequate numbers of experienced members of staff who are available to help, any threat processing is deactivated or sufficiently inhibited in order for the oxytocin-opiate-parasympathetic system to be stimulated. Staff members feel encouraged and confident, the capacity for critical thinking is retained, and it is possible to consider optimal care and compassion for the patient. Similarly, the negative impact of a difficult and unsupportive manager is reduced when there are other friendly and competent people around who act as signs of safeness for each other because they understand the situation and are able to support each other and provide valued counsel when circumstances are challenging.

Focus box 4.3   Features of safety and of being sufficiently safe

There is an absence of threat, or any threat present is reduced by or compensated for by signs of safeness

Activity of the threat processing system is suppressed but immediately available if required

Are both conditions that allow for oxytocin-opiate-parasympathetic system stimulation

---

The healthcare worker: Expressing compassion towards patients

In order for compassion to be appropriately enacted, it is necessary for the healthcare worker to feel sufficiently safe. Additionally, feeling confident in one's own skills as a healthcare professional and enjoying being of service to others can all help to bring the oxytocin-opiate-parasympathetic system 'online'. This then supports the capacity to be alert, attentive and attuned to the welfare of another human in need and engage in compassionate responding. Conveying intentional and powerful bio-behavioural signals of safety and care, encoded in speech, facial expression and bodily movement, help to build feelings of safety and connection whilst simultaneously stimulating the oxytocin-opiate-parasympathetic circuitry of the patient in turn. This mutually influencing effect results in a healthy physiological state for both the patient and the healthcare worker, and there can be a simultaneous emotional experience of 'presence and connection' between the two participants that may be experienced as compassion by the patient.

Compassionate care and contact can also provide significant comfort for patients and personal satisfaction for professionals when curative treatment is not possible (Chochinov, 2023). Importantly, the healthcare worker is present and available for the patient, and there is no undue preoccupation with self-focused feelings. In particular, a skilled healthcare worker in a calm and steady state arising from oxytocin-opiate-parasympathetic activation is able to provide a respectful 'honouring' of the integrity of the experience of suffering or vulnerability. The impulse to rush to 'fix' what may not be fixable or to offer meaningless platitudes is minimised, as is the inadvertent engendering of shame in the patient, as the healthcare worker is seen and felt to find the presence and needs of the patient in front of them, in some way intolerable.

Focus box 4.4   Key features of emotional co-regulation

Emotional co-regulation and feelings of 'presence and connection' can be experienced as compassion

Bio-behavioural signalling implicit in verbal and non-verbal communication provides the means for emotional co-regulation

Emotional co-regulation can be a mutually influencing process between members of the healthcare workforce and their patients

---

Trauma-sensitive care and compassion

Whilst it is essential to provide trauma-sensitive care within health services, to understand the relationship of safety to compassion as one that is limited to trauma sensitivity is a partial view. Compassion within the context of healthcare is necessarily trauma-sensitive but extends beyond the commitment to recognise and mitigate the effects of trauma in order to avoid re-traumatisation (Berring et al., 2024). Instead, this is an understanding of compassion that necessarily takes safety into account but one that is inclusive of an approach that intentionally promotes states of healing and restoration in patients and well-being in the workforce.

Summary points

Both skilled emotional co-regulation competencies for health-related fear and shame *and* any other profession-specific competencies required for the care of the patient are essential for patients to be safe and to experience compassion

Shame or the prospect of serious illness are potent triggers for the threat processing system

References

Berring, L. L., Holm, T., Hansen, J. P., Delcomyn, C. L., Søndergaard, R., & Hvidhjelm, J. (2024). Implementing trauma-informed care—settings, definitions, interventions, measures, and implementation across settings: A scoping review. In *Healthcare (Switzerland)* (Vol. 12, Issue 9). Multidisciplinary Digital Publishing Institute (MDPI). https://doi.org/10.3390/healthcare12090908

Chochinov, H. M. (2023). Intensive caring: Reminding patients they matter. In *Journal of Clinical Oncology* (Vol. 41, Issue 16, pp. 2884–2887). Lippincott Williams and Wilkins. https://doi.org/10.1200/JCO.23.00042

Dolezal, L. (2022). Shame anxiety, stigma and clinical encounters. *Journal of Evaluation in Clinical Practice, 28*(5), 854–860. https://doi.org/10.1111/jep.13744

Ferrari, M., Dal Cin, M., & Steele, M. (2017). Self-compassion is associated with optimum self-care behaviour, medical outcomes and psychological well-being in a cross-sectional sample of adults with diabetes. *Diabetic Medicine, 34*(11), 1546–1553. https://doi.org/10.1111/dme.13451

Gilbert, P. (2007). Evolved minds and compassion. In P. Gilbert & R. L. Leahy (Eds.), *The Therapeutic Relationship in the Cognitive Behavioral Psychotherapies* (First edition, pp. 106–142). Routledge.

Gilbert, P. (2014). The origins and nature of compassion focused therapy. *British Journal of Clinical Psychology, 53*(1), 6–41. https://doi.org/10.1111/bjc.12043

Gilbert, P. (2020). Compassion: From its evolution to a psychotherapy. *Frontiers in Psychology, 11*(December). https://doi.org/10.3389/fpsyg.2020.586161

Halifax, J. (2012). A heuristic model of enactive compassion. In *Current Opinion in Supportive and Palliative Care* (Vol. 6, Issue 2, pp. 228–235). https://doi.org/10.1097/SPC.0b013e3283530fbe

Halifax, J. (2013). G.R.A.C.E. for nurses: Cultivating compassion in nurse/patient interactions. *Journal of Nursing Education and Practice, 4*(1). https://doi.org/10.5430/jnep.v4n1p121

Heinze, K., Suwanabol, P. A., Vitous, C. A., Abrahamse, P., Gibson, K., Lansing, B., & Mody, L. (2020). A survey of patient perspectives on approach to health care: Focus on physician competency and compassion. *Journal of Patient Experience, 7*(6), 1044–1053. https://doi.org/10.1177/2374373520968447

Jaeb, M. A., & Pecanac, K. E. (2024). Shame in patient-health professional encounters: A scoping review. In *International Journal of Mental Health Nursing*. John Wiley and Sons Inc. https://doi.org/10.1111/inm.13323

MacDonald, J., & Morley, I. (2001). Shame and non-disclosure: A study of the emotional isolation of people referred for psychotherapy. *British Journal of Medical Psychology, 74*(1), 1–21. https://doi.org/10.1348/000711201160731

National Institute for Health and Social Care Excellence. (2021, June 21). *Clinical Guideline 138. Patient experience in adult NHS services: improving the experience of care for people using adult NHS services for the patient.* NICE Guideline 138 Experience Which Outlines the General Expectation of NHS Care: 1 Guidance | Patient Experience in Adult NHS Services: Improving the Experience of Care for People Using Adult NHS Services | Guidance | NICE. https://www.nice.org.uk/guidance/cg138/chapter/1-Guidance#knowing-the-patient-as-an-individual

Perry, B. (2008). Why exemplary oncology nurses seem to avoid compassion fatigue. *Canadian Oncology Nursing Journal = Revue Canadienne de Nursing Oncologique, 18*(2), 87–99. https://doi.org/10.5737/1181912x1828792

Phillips, W. J., & Hine, D. W. (2021). Self-compassion, physical health, and health behaviour: a meta-analysis. *Health Psychology Review, 15*(1), 113–139. https://doi.org/10.1080/17437199.2019.1705872

Porges, S. W. (2017). Vagal pathways: Portals to compassion. In E. M. Seppala, E. Simon-Thomas, S. L. Brown, M. C. Worline, C. D. Cameron, & J. R. Doty (Eds.), *The Oxford Handbook of Compassion Science* (pp. 189–202). Oxford University Press.

Sinclair, S., McClement, S., Raffin-Bouchal, S., Hack, T. F., Hagen, N. A., McConnell, S., & Chochinov, H. M. (2016). Compassion in health care: An empirical model. *Journal of Pain and Symptom Management, 51*(2), 193–203. https://doi.org/10.1016/j.jpainsymman.2015.10.009

Thayer, J. F., Yamamoto, S. S., & Brosschot, J. F. (2010). The relationship of autonomic imbalance, heart rate variability and cardiovascular disease risk factors. In *International Journal of Cardiology* (Vol. 141, Issue 2, pp. 122–131). https://doi.org/10.1016/j.ijcard.2009.09.543

Thienprayoon, R., Sinclair, S., Lown, B. A., Pestian, T., Awtrey, E., Winick, N., & Kanov, J. (2022). Organizational compassion: Ameliorating healthcare worker's suffering and burnout. *Journal of Wellness, 4*(1), 3–5. https://doi.org/10.55504/2578-9333.1122

Trzeciak, S., & Mazzarelli, A. (2019a). The physiological health benefits of compassion. In *Compassionomics. The Revolutionary Scientific Evidence that Caring Makes a Difference* (First edition, pp. 47–90). Studer Group, LLC.

Trzeciak, S., & Mazzarelli, A. (2019b). The psychological health benefits of compassion. In *Compassionomics. The Revolutionary Scientific Evidence that Caring Makes a Difference* (First edition, pp. 91–124). Studer Group, LLC.

West, M. A. (2021). *Compassionate Leadership*. Swirling Leaf Press.

5   Barriers to compassion in healthcare

This chapter explores some of the common barriers to compassion in healthcare that have been identified. Both uniquely human factors, along with collective and organisational factors, that either act in isolation or interact and that can contribute to a lack of compassion in healthcare systems are explored.

Lack of knowledge

The influence of ethnicity on compassion is under-explored (Goetz et al., 2010), and this lack of knowledge may be a barrier to compassion in itself. In particular, studies of the influence of ethnicity in both receiving and offering care to people of the same or differing ethnic backgrounds and cultural practices remain rare (Singh et al., 2018). The degree to which people want to avoid feeling negative and base their own compassionate responding on their own preferences is thought to vary between cultures, as are other features of compassion relating to the conceptualisation, expression and experience of compassion (Koopmann-Holm & Tsai, 2017; Seow et al., 2024). Whilst there are also similarities in compassion across cultures (Armstrong, 2011; Koopmann-Holm & Tsai, 2017), it is important that what are apparently shared ethnic or cultural practices or beliefs do not lead to assumptions about what may or may not constitute compassion in practice for any given individual (Singh et al., 2018).

Lack of safety

When healthcare workers do not feel safe at work, either physically or psychologically, or both, attention becomes more focused on the need to establish safety for oneself, and so it reduces the capacity to focus on the needs of sick and vulnerable patients. Consequently, the capacity to embody compassion is impeded if not curtailed. The

DOI: 10.4324/9781003427247-5

available psychological capital and resources for safe, effective and creative team-working are eroded (West, 2021b), and metabolic resources otherwise used to support well-being and flourishing in the workforce are diverted to defend and protect functions. All of the barriers below represent a lack of safety in one form or another for either patients or members of the workforce.

De-humanisation, objectification and 'othering'

The degree of similarity and emotional compatibility shared with others is known to be a powerful influence on the expression of compassion (Goetz et al., 2010) and arises from an evolutionary past in which small groups of family members and familiar people represented the main source of safety. People who are perceived as very poor, homeless or as having problems with substance misuse may be subject to disgust and consequent 'de-humanisation' whilst people who appear to be very successful and with apparently few challenges in life can be envied and subject to 'objectification' (Fiske, 2009, p. 31).

Either way, the individuals concerned are seen as less than human in some way and, as a result, are less likely to be regarded with empathy or to be offered compassion. Patients classified as having a low social economic status have also been shown to report the experience of low empathy from healthcare professionals, along with a trend for the experience of low empathy to be reported by people of mixed race and other ethnicities, in contrast to those classified as white (Roberts et al., 2021). These responses, when they occur, however, are thought to be automatic and unconscious (Harris & Fiske, 2007), and whilst this automaticity does not constitute a personal failing, it is important to know about them and to use more conscious processing to overcome them (Fiske, 2009) particularly in the context of healthcare.

Patients and professionals

Within healthcare, harsh judgement as an impediment to compassion can be common. People with morbid obesity are often judged for their weight, and their motivation to lose weight is sometimes questioned, despite the evident suffering and considerable health risks involved (Hughes et al., 2021; Trzeciak & Mazzarelli, 2019). People with facial disfigurement also appear to provoke less empathy on a neurological level, as part of a process of unconscious bias (Hartung et al., 2019).

Patients who did not follow self-care instructions were experienced as depleting and less deserving of care than other people (Tierney et al., 2017), and those who are judged to be ungrateful are less likely to be offered compassion in response (Pavlova et al., 2022). Patients who were experienced as difficult or non-compliant, or who were judged as responsible for their own illness, also all attracted lower compassion scores when rated by medical students (Wang et al., 2022). People judged as difficult were also reported to thwart efforts at compassion from healthcare workers in dental clinics (Alvenfors et al., 2022) as well as in other settings (Baguley et al., 2020).

The 'hierarchical imbalance of the clinical relationship' (DasGupta, 2008, p. 981) may also impede a compassionate response on an individual level. It has been observed that some healthcare encounters between professionals and patients appear to have a dual function. On the one hand, the healthcare professional is required to engage in a delicate conversational process conveying power, authority and expert status (Nettleton, 1995), but on the other, there is a requirement that both participants co-create feelings of safety and connection in the name of compassion. This delicate process, when disrupted by a refusal to acquiesce to the lesser role on the part of the patient, can lead to a wrangling of control over the encounter (Nettleton, 1995). Consequently, opportunities for compassion are lost because cooperation rather than competition is needed to co-create a safe relationship as the basis for compassion.

Racism

Racism is inherently uncompassionate and unsafe for patients and staff. Racism is known to be a scourge throughout healthcare systems worldwide (Benjamin et al., 2022; Fitzgerald & Hurst, 2017; Harris et al., 2024; McLane et al., 2022; NHS England, 2022a) as well as enervating societal strength more broadly (Benjamin et al., 2022). Racism adversely impacts both patients and the workforce, manifesting at both the institutional and individual level and is often a contributing factor in high-profile failures of care (e.g., Ockenden, 2022).

Racism itself has been described as a pernicious process of 'de-humanising societal valuation' (Professor C P Jones, quoted in Samarasekera, 2023, p. 811) and one that may be internalised by those people who are persistently subject to it (Jones, 2000). Along with other structural factors supporting the status quo, racism remains a fundamental basis of health inequity (Samarasekera, 2023) that has yet to be effectively addressed (Wu et al., 2023). Meanwhile, biological mechanisms for the harms caused by microaggressions as well as overt racism specifically, are becoming more clearly understood (Dong et al., 2022; Juster et al., 2010) as a stressor that can adversely impact staff well-being in health care settings.

Focus box 5.1   Bias and othering

The human mind is subject to automatic and unconscious processes of bias and 'othering'

Patients who are subject to bias are at considerable risk of poorer health outcomes

Knowing about and reducing harmful processes of automaticity and reactivity that disadvantage some patients and some members of the healthcare workforce is important

---

Violence and aggression

Violence in the healthcare workplace appears to occur the world over (Vento et al., 2020) and has been found to include sexual violence perpetrated by and on members of the healthcare workforce (Begeny et al., 2023). Each assault on a healthcare worker activates the threat processing system and provokes a 'fight or flight' response in the moment or sometimes a 'freeze' response, depending upon the threat severity. It is not unusual for healthcare workers in particular areas, for example, in ER or community settings, to be exposed to the repeated risk of assault when sufficient safety is not able to be guaranteed. Unfortunately, either a personal experience of violence or of seeing others assaulted can re-tune the autonomic nervous system of the individual concerned to become increasingly sensitive to threat, and for some members of the workforce, such experiences can lead to the development of Post-traumatic Stress Disorder.

Social mentalities: Ancient psychologies of mind in contemporary settings

Inherited psychologies and tendencies of mind called social mentalities (Gilbert, 2009a) are present in everyone. Originally designed to support behaviour and relationships conducive to survival and kinship in the context of very different societal structures and environmental conditions, they continue to operate as a feature of relationships in contemporary settings (Gilbert, 2020, 2021). So, for example, there is a social mentality that organises thinking and behaviour around competition and another that organises on the basis of finding groups of people like oneself to enable feelings of community. These normal and useful ways of functioning are all still part of an acquired landscape of human psychology that is shaped by a shared evolutionary past and that affects behaviour in the present. Social mentalities are not, however, without their complexities and can cause problems if there is a lack of awareness of their potential effects in newer contexts.

A social mentality concerned with care giving and compassion and that is conducive to good healthcare may be eclipsed by one less conducive to good healthcare, given pressurised conditions, and this can then result in harm to both patients and colleagues. Intensely competitive and rivalrous relationships anywhere in a healthcare system can lead to dysfunction in services for patients and unhappiness for members of the workforce directly impacted. Whilst these, amongst other inherited features of human nature, are not a cause for blame, these too become at least in part, a personal responsibility to be addressed because of their potential to harm others (Gilbert, 2009a).

Unfortunately, it is the case that healthcare organisations are sometimes structured in ways that create division and discord by actively cultivating competition for resources or rewards (Gilbert, 2009a). Over time, these processes may become normalised, and any balance or perspective on what constitutes a compassionate workplace is lost to a strong competitive ethos (Gilbert, 2009b). Time pressures and competing demands, for example, paper work, and a culture of 'threat' from within organisations themselves and, at times, patients, are all described as impeding compassionate care, and this refrain is repeated many times over (Dixon-Woods et al., 2014; Pavlova et al., 2022; Rydon-Grange, 2018; Thienprayoon et al., 2022; e.g., Tierney et al., 2017; Wang et al., 2022).

Institutional, organisational and team factors

Hospitals are very hierarchical institutions with much in-built social comparison (Michalec et al., 2024), and strongly enforced relationships of deference to those with power and in authority may play out in harmful ways in any setting (Gilbert, 2009a). In hospitals, for example, it is known that strongly hierarchical leadership at the team level can stifle compassionate communication between staff and the capacity to respond effectively to the suffering of patients (Kanaris, 2023). Hierarchy is also known to be a contributor to disrespectful behaviour between staff (Leape et al., 2012), and it has been suggested that extreme competitiveness in healthcare leadership may be a significant barrier to a compassionate organisation (Basran et al., 2019).

In laboratory experiments it has been demonstrated that if money concerns are uppermost, the degree of empathy experienced and capacity to express compassion are both reduced (Molinsky et al., 2012). Furthermore, working in systems that prioritise money and efficiency over compassionate working for staff is harmful and unlikely to achieve desired outcomes for patients (Pavlova et al., 2023) as well as being associated with lower levels of compassion in medical trainees (Wang et al., 2022).

Clearly, it is not the responsibility of individual members of the workforce alone to try to address organisational shortcomings, but compassionate leadership across the health and social care sectors is vital in ensuring that each individual in an organisation can take their place and play their part within a growing movement committed to improving compassionate care (West, 2021a).

Bullying, harassment and incivility

Bullying, harassment and incivility are each socially nuanced forms of intimidation and anti-social behaviour that evoke submissive and fearful responses, and indeed, they are intended to do so. They represent, in essence, an indicator to the victim that they are regarded as inferior in some way to the perpetrator, and such an unfavourable social comparison is a potent trigger for the threat processing system. There is reduced sense of safety, albeit psychological, and as a result any desire or capacity to behave compassionately or creatively becomes stifled as people become preoccupied with defending or protecting themselves (West, 2021b).

Bullying, harassment and incivility is known to play out across different professional groups and in many healthcare systems (e.g., Mammen et al., 2023; Naylor et al., 2022; Santosa et al., 2023). Healthcare workers from black and minority ethnic groups continue to be at increased risk of bullying, abuse and harassment overall when compared to people from other ethnic groups (NHS England, 2022a), as are people with disabilities when compared to those without disabilities (NHS England, 2022b). Perpetrators of anti-social interpersonal behaviour include patients, relatives and members of the public, but it is clear that staff play a part in this too (NHS England, 2022b).

Being the target of rudeness or witnessing rudeness between colleagues at work is known to have negative effects on both individual and team performance, including a degradation of the quality of work (Porath & Pearson, 2015). Furthermore, there is ample evidence of the detrimental effect of anti-social behaviour in healthcare systems on both patients and staff more generally (Lever et al., 2019; Martin & Zadinsky, 2022; Sylvester, 2023; Woo & Kim, 2020).

Summary points

> Individual factors can interact with organisational factors to increase barriers to compassionate care

Some social mentalities can be harmful if they go unnoticed and unchecked

Healthcare organisations can be organised in ways that reward competition and rivalry

Psychological and physical safety are needed to support workforce well-being in order to provide compassionate care for patients

References

Alvenfors, A., Velic, M., Marklund, B., Kylén, S., Lingström, P., & Bernson,J. (2022). "Difficult" dental patients: A grounded theory study of dental staff's experiences. *BDJ Open, 8*(1), 24. https://doi.org/10.1038/s41405-022-00115-7

Armstrong, K. (2011). *Twelve Steps to a Compassionate Life* (First edition). The Bodley Head.

Baguley, S. I., Dev, V., Fernando, A. T., & Consedine, N. S. (2020). How do health professionals maintain compassion over time? Insights from a study of compassion in health. *Frontiers in Psychology, 11*(December), 1–11. https://doi.org/10.3389/fpsyg.2020.564554

Basran, J., Pires, C., Matos, M., McEwan, K., & Gilbert, P. (2019). Styles of leadership, fears of compassion, and competing to avoid inferiority. *Frontiers in Psychology, 9*(January). https://doi.org/10.3389/fpsyg.2018.02460

Begeny, C. T., Arshad, H., Cuming, T., Dhariwal, D. K., Fisher, R. A., Franklin, M. D., Jackson, P. M., McLachlan, G. M., Searle, R. H., & Newlands, C. (2023). Sexual harassment, sexual assault and rape by colleagues in the surgical workforce, and how women and men are living different realities: Observational study using NHS population-derived weights. *British Journal of Surgery, 110*(11), 1518–1526. https://doi.org/10.1093/bjs/znad242

Benjamin, G. C., Jones, C. P., & Davis Moss, R. (2022). Editorial: Racism as a public health crisis: From declaration to action. In *Frontiers in Public Health* (Vol. 10, pp. 1–2). Frontiers Media S.A. https://doi.org/10.3389/fpubh.2022.893804

Curtis, P., & Wood, C. (2023). *Martha's Rule. A New Policy to Amplify Patient Voice and Improve Safety in Hospitals*. www.demos.co.uk

DasGupta, S. (2008). Narrative humility. In *Lancet* (Vol. 371, Issue 9617, pp. 980–981). https://doi.org/10.1016/S0140-6736(08)60440-7

Dixon-Woods, M., Baker, R., Charles, K., Dawson, J., Jerzembek, G., Martin, G., McCarthy, I., McKee, L., Minion, J., Ozieranski, P., Willars, J., Wilkie, P., & West, M. (2014). Culture and behaviour in the English National Health Service: Overview of lessons from a large multimethod study. *BMJ Quality and Safety, 23*(2), 106–115. https://doi.org/10.1136/bmjqs-2013-001947

Dong, T. S., Gee, G. C., Beltran-Sanchez, H., Wang, M., Osadchiy, V., Kilpatrick, L. A., Chen, Z., Subramanyam, V., Zhang, Y., Guo, Y., Labus, J. S., Naliboff, B., Cole, S., Zhang, X., Mayer, E. A., & Gupta, A. (2022). How discrimination gets under the skin: Biological determinants of discrimination associated with dysregulation of the brain-gut microbiome system and psychological symptoms. *Biological Psychiatry*. https://doi.org/10.1016/j.biopsych.2022.10.011

Fiske, S. T. (2009). From dehumanization and objectification to rehumanization: Neuroimaging studies on the building blocks of empathy. *Annals of the New York Academy of Sciences, 1167*, 31–34. https://doi.org/10.1111/j.1749-6632.2009.04544.x

Fitzgerald, C., & Hurst, S. (2017). Implicit bias in healthcare professionals: A systematic review. *BMC Medical Ethics*, *18*(1). https://doi.org/10.1186/s12910-017-0179-8

Gilbert, P. (2009a). Placing ourselves in the flow of life. In *The Compassionate Mind: A New Approach to Life's Challenges*. (First edition, pp. 79–122). New Harbinger Publications, Inc.

Gilbert, P. (2009b). The pleasures and contentment of life: The two types of good feelings and your compassionate mind. In *The Compassionate Mind. A New Approach to Life's Challenges* (First edition, pp. 149–180). New Harbinger Publications Ltd.

Gilbert, P. (2020). Compassion: From Its Evolution to a Psychotherapy. *Frontiers in Psychology*, *11*(December). https://doi.org/10.3389/fpsyg.2020.586161

Gilbert, P. (2021). Creating a compassionate world: Addressing the conflicts between sharing and caring versus controlling and holding evolved strategies. *Frontiers in Psychology*, *11*(February). https://doi.org/10.3389/fpsyg.2020.582090

Goetz, J. L., Keltner, D., & Simon-Thomas, E. (2010). Compassion: An evolutionary analysis and empirical review. *Psychological Bulletin*, *136*(3), 351–374. https://doi.org/10.1037/a0018807

Harris, L. T., & Fiske, S. T. (2007). Social groups that elicit disgust are differentially processed in mPFC. *Social Cognitive and Affective Neuroscience*, *2*(1), 45–51. https://doi.org/10.1093/scan/nsl037

Harris, R., Cormack, D., Waa, A., Edwards, R., & Stanley, J. (2024). The impact of racism on subsequent healthcare use and experiences for adult New Zealanders: A prospective cohort study. *BMC Public Health*, *24*(1). https://doi.org/10.1186/s12889-023-17603-6

Hartung, F., Jamrozik, A., Rosen, M. E., Aguirre, G., Sarwer, D. B., & Chatterjee, A. (2019). Behavioural and neural responses to facial disfigurement. *Scientific Reports*, *9*(1), 8021. https://doi.org/10.1038/s41598-019-44408-8

Hughes, C. A., Ahern, A. L., Kasetty, H., McGowan, B. M., Parretti, H. M., Vincent, A., & Halford, J. C. G. (2021). Changing the narrative around obesity in the UK: A survey of people with obesity and healthcare professionals from the ACTION-IO study. *BMJ Open*, *11*(6). https://doi.org/10.1136/bmjopen-2020-045616

Jones, C. P. (2000). Levels of racism: A theoretic framework and a gardener's tale. *American Journal of Public Health*, *90*(8), 1212–1215.

Juster, R. P., McEwen, B. S., & Lupien, S. J. (2010). Allostatic load biomarkers of chronic stress and impact on health and cognition. *Neuroscience and Biobehavioral Reviews*, *35*(1), 2–16. https://doi.org/10.1016/j.neubiorev.2009.10.002

Kanaris, C. (2023). Mind the power gap: How hierarchical leadership in healthcare is a risk to patient safety. In *Journal of Child Health Care* (Vol. 27, Issue 3, pp. 319–322). SAGE Publications Inc. https://doi.org/10.1177/13674935231196197

Koopmann-Holm, B., & Tsai, J. L. (2017). The cultural shaping of compassion. In E. Seppala, E. Simon-Thomas, S. L. Brown, M. C. Worline, D. C. Cameron, & J. R. Doty (Eds.), *The Oxford Handbook of Compassion Science* (First edition, pp. 273–283). Oxford University Press.

Leape, L. L., Shore, M. F., Dienstag, J. L., Mayer, R. J., Edgman-Levitan, S., Meyer, G. S., & Healy, G. B. (2012). Perspective: A culture of respect, Part 1: The nature and causes of disrespectful behavior by physicians. In *Academic Medicine* (Vol. 87,

Issue 7, pp. 845–852). Lippincott Williams and Wilkins. https://doi.org/10.1097/ACM.0b013e318258338d

Lever, I., Dyball, D., Greenberg, N., & Stevelink, S. A. M. (2019). Health consequences of bullying in the healthcare workplace: A systematic review. In *Journal of Advanced Nursing* (Vol. 75, Issue 12, pp. 3195–3209). Blackwell Publishing Ltd. https://doi.org/10.1111/jan.13986

Mammen, B. N., Lam, L., & Hills, D. (2023). Newly qualified graduate nurses' experiences of workplace incivility in healthcare settings: An integrative review. In *Nurse Education in Practice* (Vol. 69). Elsevier Ltd. https://doi.org/10.1016/j.nepr.2023.103611

Martin, L. D., & Zadinsky, J. K. (2022). Frequency and outcomes of workplace incivility in healthcare: A scoping review of the literature. In *Journal of Nursing Management* (Vol. 30, Issue 7, pp. 3496–3518). John Wiley and Sons Inc. https://doi.org/10.1111/jonm.13783

McLane, P., Mackey, L., Holroyd, B. R., Fitzpatrick, K., Healy, C., Rittenbach, K., Plume, T. B., Bill, L., Bird, A., Healy, B., Janvier, K., Louis, E., & Barnabe, C. (2022). Impacts of racism on First Nations patients' emergency care: Results of a thematic analysis of healthcare provider interviews in Alberta, Canada. *BMC Health Services Research*, *22*(1). https://doi.org/10.1186/s12913-022-08129-5

Michalec, B., Cuddy, M. M., Felix, K., Gur-Arie, R., Tilburt, J. C., & Hafferty, F. W. (2024). Positioning humility within healthcare delivery - From doctors' and nurses' perspectives. *Human Factors in Healthcare*, *5*. https://doi.org/10.1016/j.hfh.2023.100061

Molinsky, A. L., Grant, A. M., & Margolis, J. D. (2012). The bedside manner of homo economicus: How and why priming an economic schema reduces compassion. *Organizational Behavior and Human Decision Processes*, *119*(1), 27–37. https://doi.org/10.1016/j.obhdp.2012.05.001

Myers, C. G., Lu-Myers, Y., & Ghaferi, A. A. (2018). Excising the "surgeon ego" to accelerate progress in the culture of surgery. *BMJ (Online)*, *363*. https://doi.org/10.1136/bmj.k4537

Naylor, M. J., Boyes, C., & Killingback, C. (2022). "You've broken the patient": Physiotherapists' lived experience of incivility within the healthcare team - An Interpretative Phenomenological Analysis. *Physiotherapy (United Kingdom)*, *117*, 89–96. https://doi.org/10.1016/j.physio.2022.09.001

Nettleton, S. (1995). The sociology of lay-professional interactions. In *The Sociology of Health and Illness* (First edition, pp. 131–159). Polity Press.

NHS England. (2022a). NHS workforce race equality standard (WRES). 2022 data analysis report for NHS trusts. In *Be*. https://www.england.nhs.uk/publication/nhs-workforce-race-equality-standard-2022/

NHS England. (2022b). *Workforce Disability Equality Standard 2022 Data Analysis Report for NHS Trusts and Foundation Trusts*. https://www.england.nhs.uk/publication/workforce-disability-equality-standard-2022-data-analysis-report-for-nhs-trusts-and-foundation-trusts/

Ockenden, D. (2022). *Ockenden Report. Findings, Conclusions and Essential Actions from the Independent Review of Maternity Services at The Shrewsbury and Telford Hospital NHS Trust: Our Final Report*. https://www.gov.uk/government/publications/final-report-of-the-ockenden-review

Pavlova, A., Paine, S. J., Sinclair, S., O'Callaghan, A., & Considine, N. S. (2023). Working in value-discrepant environments inhibits clinicians' ability to provide compassion and reduces well-being: A cross-sectional study. *Journal of Internal Medicine, 293*(6), 704–723. https://doi.org/10.1111/joim.13615 Pavlova, A., Wang, C. X. Y., Boggiss, A. L., O'Callaghan, A., & Considine, N. S. (2022). Predictors of physician compassion, empathy, and related constructs: A systematic review. *Journal of General Internal Medicine, 37*(4), 900–911. https://doi.org/10.1007/s11606-021-07055-2

Porath, C., & Pearson, C. (2015). The price of incivility. In *HBR's 10 Must Reads. The Price of Incivility: Lack of Respect Hurts Morale - and the Bottom Line* (First edition, pp. 93–104). Harvard Business Review Press.

Roberts, B. W., Puri, N. K., Trzeciak, C. J., Mazzarelli, A. J., & Id, S. T. (2021). *Socioeconomic, Racial and Ethnic Differences in Patient Experience of Clinician Empathy: Results of a Systematic Review and Meta- Analysis.* 1–16. https://doi.org/10.1371/journal.pone.0247259

Rydon-Grange, M. (2018). Psychological perspective on compassion in modern healthcare settings. *Journal of Medical Ethics, 44*(11), 729–733. https://doi.org/10.1136/medethics-2017-104698

Samarasekera, U. (2022). Helen Hansen: Developing structural humility in medicine. *The Lancet, 399*(10340), 2007. https://doi.org/10.1016/S0140-6736(22)00931-X

Samarasekera, U. (2023). Profile. Camara Phyllis Jones: Anti-racism thought leader. *The Lancet, 401*, 811.

Santosa, K. B., Hayward, L., Matusko, N., Kubiak, C. A., Strong, A. L., Waljee, J. F., Jagsi, R., & Sandhu, G. (2023). Attributions and perpetrators of incivility in academic surgery. *Global Surgical Education - Journal of the Association for Surgical Education, 2*(1). https://doi.org/10.1007/s44186-023-00129-1

Seow, J. H., Du, H., & Koopmann-Holm, B. (2024). What is a compassionate face? Avoided negative affect explains differences between U.S. Americans and Chinese. *Cognition and Emotion*, 1–10. https://doi.org/10.1080/02699931.2024.2385708

Singh, P., King-Shier, K., & Sinclair, S. (2018). The colours and contours of compassion: A systematic review of the perspectives of compassion among ethnically diverse patients and healthcare providers. In *PLoS ONE* (Vol. 13, Issue 5). Public Library of Science. https://doi.org/10.1371/journal.pone.0197261

Sylvester, R. (2023, November 18). Toxic doctors put patients at risk, says NHS watchdog. https://www.thetimes.co.uk/article/toxic-culture-among-nhs-doctors-times-health-commission-g3ltrt7f0

Thienprayoon, R., Sinclair, S., Lown, B. A., Pestian, T., Awtrey, E., Winick, N., & Kanov, J. (2022). Organizational compassion: Ameliorating healthcare worker's suffering and burnout. *Journal of Wellness, 4*(1), 3–5. https://doi.org/10.55504/2578-9333.1122

Tierney, S., Seers, K., Tutton, E., & Reeve, J. (2017). Enabling the flow of compassionate care: A grounded theory study. *BMC Health Services Research, 17*(1), 1–12. https://doi.org/10.1186/s12913-017-2120-8

Trzeciak, S., & Mazzarelli, A. (2019). Nature versus nurture: Can we learn compassion? In *Compassionomics. The Revolutionary Scientific Evidence That Caring Makes a Difference* (First edition, pp. 263–286). Studer Group.

Vento, S., Cainelli, F., & Vallone, A. (2020). Violence against healthcare workers: A worldwide phenomenon with serious consequences. *Frontiers in Public Health, 8*. https://doi.org/10.3389/fpubh.2020.570459

Wang, C. X. Y., Pavlova, A., Boggiss, A. L., O'Callaghan, A., & Consedine, N. S. (2022). Predictors of medical students' compassion and related constructs: A systematic review. *Teaching and Learning in Medicine*, 1–12. https://doi.org/10.1080/10401334.2022.2103816

West, M. A. (2021a). *Compassionate Leadership*. Swirling Leaf Press.

West, M. A. (2021b). Compassionate team leadership and psychological safety. In *Compassionate Leadership* (pp. 87–109). Swirling Leaf Press.

Woo, C. H., & Kim, C. (2020). Impact of workplace incivility on compassion competence of Korean nurses: Moderating effect of psychological capital. *Journal of Nursing Management*. https://doi.org/10.1111/jonm.12982

Wu, A. W., Vincent, C., Øvretveit, J., Mair, A., Buckle, P., Garcia Elorrio, E., Bellandi, T., Letaief, M., Ushiro, S., & Koizumi, S. (2023). Gaps in patient safety: Areas that need our attention. In *Journal of Patient Safety and Risk Management* (Vol. 28, Issue 6, pp. 246–252). SAGE Publications Ltd. https://doi.org/10.1177/25160435231218489

6 Patient and healthcare workers' views on compassion

This chapter draws out a small number of themes repeatedly identified within patient and healthcare workers descriptions of compassion. Looked at from the perspective of the function of compassion, these descriptions appear to endorse the view of emotional co-regulation as key to the expression and experience of compassion. This chapter also speaks to the role of the nurse in compassion, along with common humanity and humility in compassionate contact with patients.

No bigger picture

Much of the work exploring compassion from a patient perspective has focused on people receiving end-of-life care or cancer treatment and on the role of nurses and doctors. There has been less research conducted with other groups, for example, with people who have a psychiatric illness, those with sensory impairments, or in more varied healthcare settings. There is a paucity of research involving non-clinicians, although patients not infrequently mention the importance of small acts of compassion from hospitality, housekeeping or other staff that they come into contact with in healthcare facilities. As a result, what is available is likely to contribute to an imbalanced or partial picture that may be missing important similarities and differences in the experience and expression of compassion across a range of health and social care settings and for different groups of people including those of different ethnicities and cultures.

Nurses and compassion

Nurses are sometimes seen as the prime repository for compassion within healthcare (Bivins et al., 2017; Menzies, 1960). Compassion is an expectation enshrined in practice guidelines (Nursing and Midwifery Council, 2018) and a quality of care that is often afforded a high profile in relation to nursing when compared to other professions. Experts in the field of compassion have also acknowledged the accomplishments

DOI: 10.4324/9781003427247-6

of their nursing colleagues in providing compassionate care for patients and hold them up as exemplars (see dedication Trzeciak & Mazzarelli, 2019a), whilst other researchers have referenced possible differences of training culture and emphasis on compassion between the medical and nursing professions (Dev et al., 2019).

Nurses may also be held more accountable than other professions when there is found to be a lack of compassionate care. Nurses in the UK for example, were singled out, along with their systems of governance, for harsh criticism in failing to provide compassionate care for patients (Francis, 2013), in spite of enormously complex failures at all organisational levels, including those of medical leadership (Holmes, 2013), that may well also have contributed to care lacking in compassion (Tierney et al., 2019).

From the perspective of Porges's description of the function of compassion, however, it appears that it may be the role of the nurse, above all other professions, that most closely aligns with *bearing professional witness to the suffering and vulnerability of patients without triggering feelings of health-related shame.*

Whilst nurses have a variety of other diverse and extended roles in relation to the care of patients, for example, those in advanced nurse practitioner positions, it is nurses and healthcare assistants who routinely care for those who are most vulnerable. It is also almost exclusively nurses or healthcare assistants who are the first point of contact and called upon to attend to patients who have been incontinent or who have vomited when they are due to be seen by other healthcare professionals. Nurses, it seems, in many settings are repeatedly called upon to bear professional witness to people in varying states of acute vulnerability and potentially at risk of health-related shame. In addition to any other profession-specific or role-related competencies required, this particular dimension of care demands effective relational and emotional co-regulation skills. This is firstly in order to avoid activating the threat processing system in vulnerable people, and secondly to stimulate the oxytocin-opiate-parasympathetic circuitry to provide feelings of comfort, safety and encouragement for patients in the most difficult of situations.

Such intimate work is often regarded as lowly in nature, however, and tends to be much less valued and attract less favourable remuneration in comparison with care that requires more technical proficiency (Dev et al., 2019; Kelly et al., 2018; Nettleton, 1995). As is attested to by an emerging evidence-base, however, it appears to be the case that the relational skills honed when caring for people at their most vulnerable have a valuable and dual role. The skills involved not only promote healing and restoration in patients, but simultaneously, can play a part in supporting individual wellbeing by allowing healthcare workers to feel connected to the value and meaning of their work (Perry, 2008).

'Being present' and feeling connected as compassion

There is abundant evidence attesting to the fact that the key ingredient of compassionate care is the relationship between the patient and healthcare provider (Chochinov, 2023; Malenfant et al., 2022; Sinclair et al., 2017). To be present with, and available for patients, is a necessary precondition for compassion to be experienced and critical to a good patient experience (Gillespie & Reader, 2021). Patients are easily able to tell when the people who are caring for them are preoccupied and only partially attentive and are greatly appreciative when healthcare workers are able to offer their presence: 'They're actually there, you can see that they're there in mind and body, they're not off somewhere else' (Sinclair, McClement, et al., 2016, p. 200 Participant 25).

Patients also understand exactly what it is that healthcare workers need to do in order for them to feel that they have received compassionate care. 'They have to learn how to be in tune with people in the moment' (Sinclair, Torres, et al., 2016, p. 6), or the healthcare worker should be seen to be 'trying to get alongside' the person that they are caring for (Bond et al., 2022, p. 34). When healthcare professionals let people know of the intention to 'accompany' them on their healthcare journey (Trzeciak & Mazzarelli, 2019b) or take the time to be seated and take their place beside them (Patel et al., 2019) in a way that indicates 'availability', care and attention, patients are comforted and feel themselves to be the recipients of compassion.

Patients appear to seek some sense of connection, or even closeness, with the people who care for them (Lown et al., 2011; Sinclair et al., 2017), and skilled staff understand and appreciate the importance of providing connection as part of compassionate care (Perry, 2008; Tierney et al., 2019). There is a sense of authenticity in these sorts of experiences of closeness and connection between health professionals and their patients (Baguley et al., 2020; Bond et al., 2022; Perry, 2008) and often a sense of relief on the part of patients, perhaps because of the way that health-related shame and health-related fear can both be very effective channels for isolation.

Patients' descriptions of the quality of a relationship that is valued appear to 'give voice' to what is an embodied and subjective human experience. Verbatim reports from patients refer to a 'heartfelt connection' as part of the experience of compassion (Durkin et al., 2019, p. 1386; Way & Tracy, 2012), whilst others note the process of scanning nurses faces for signs of anger and harshness or softness and receptivity (Bond et al., 2022, p. 4031, Participant 2; Younas et al., 2023). The behavioural vectors or bio-behavioural signals displayed by healthcare professionals and involved in emotional co-regulation as identified by (Patel et al 2019) have also been described clearly by patients: 'Their demeanour, their body language, how they speak to you, their tone of voice, the eye contact that they make with you. I think those are the primary indicators (Sinclair, McClement, et al., 2016, p. 199 Participant 45).

The felt sense of compassion has been described variously as 'connection on a human-human level' (Bond et al., 2022, p. 33) or the healthcare professional 'giving the feeling' (Bond et al., 2022, p. 33) or of compassion being linked specifically with a sense of calm and safety (Bond et al., 2022) or of a reduction in anxiety (Trzeciak & Mazzarelli, 2019b). Similarly, the essence of compassion may be experienced as a transmission of sorts: 'I can feel people's compassion. 'You feel it coming off them' (Sinclair, McClement, et al., 2016, p. 196, Participant 27) or 'I would have to say, I know it intuitively' (Sinclair, McClement, et al., 2016, p. 196 Participant 47). Each of these descriptions reflect a visceral sense of relationship conducted through mutually influencing bio-behavioural signalling systems that work to dampen the threat processing system and stimulate the oxytocin-opiate-parasympathetic system in order to co-create safe and healthy connections between patients and the people that care for them.

Compassion as brief action

Compassion is a behaviour or action-based (unlike empathic concern) and it can be effectively and intentionally conveyed by *how something is done* rather than just what is done (Perry, 2009; Singh et al., 2018). It has been observed that some nurses have the ability to convey compassion in the briefest of moments and with the smallest of gestures (Bramley & Matiti, 2014; Malenfant et al., 2022; Schwartz, 1995), and that, furthermore, the brevity and simplicity of such acts can be experienced just as powerfully as more elaborate demonstrations of compassion (Younas et al., 2023). A 40-second speech-based intervention by doctors has also been found to convey compassion effectively in a routine clinical setting (Trzeciak & Mazzarelli, 2019b), and it is also known that compassion can be easily conveyed through small 'every day' actions, essential for basic care (Perry, 2009). It is important to note, however, that sufficient time is required to carry out basic care in an attentive and attuned fashion, and some researchers have found this basic need to be sadly lacking in contemporary healthcare systems (Tierney et al., 2019).

Focus box 6.1   Features of the experience of compassion as reported by patients

Intuitive
Visceral
Presence
Connection
Conveyed by the quality of action (how something is done)

Common humanity

Connecting with a sense of common humanity in order to facilitate compassionate care is thought to be essential for healthcare workers (Thienprayoon et al., 2022), and it has also been said that compassion requires that the healthcare provider '…engage and relate to suffering from a place of shared humanity' by other experts in the field (Sinclair, McClement, et al., 2016, p. 202). The understanding of a shared humanity is also a commonly identified theme in some definitions of compassion (e.g., Jazaieri et al., 2013; Strauss et al., 2016), and in particular, understanding the ubiquity of the vulnerability to suffering has been found to help some healthcare workers to retain a compassionate stance over time (Baguley et al., 2020). Somewhat similarly, the personal experience of suffering in healthcare workers has also been reported as supporting the capacity to respond compassionately in a professional context (Dev et al., 2019; Singh et al., 2018).

In a palliative care setting, patients urged the importance of a greater understanding of common humanity by staff in relation to compassion (Selman et al., 2018), and in another study, patients with complex care needs suggested that staff members try to understand their patients as simply other varied expressions of humanity in the face of any difficulties in feeling connected with them (Younas et al., 2023). Sympathy was described by patients in a palliative care setting as something that was not focused on their needs and placed unwanted distance between them and their caregivers, and overall, was experienced as deleterious to their health (Sinclair et al., 2017). It appears that if healthcare professionals remain too distant from their patients, their capacity to co-create a relationship that acts as a vehicle for compassionate co-regulation and connection is compromised. This is skilled and sensitive work, however, as there are also problems for members of the workforce if the nature of the compassionate relationship becomes confused with an unhelpful process of over-identification and fusion with the suffering of others.

Humility

Humility has been described as a means of preserving compassionate care within the context of difficult interactions with patients (Tierney et al., 2017), and patients have linked humility and compassion. Patients report appreciating humility when nurses are unable to answer their questions (Sinclair, Torres, et al., 2016) and when they avoid 'talking down' to the people in their care (Younas et al., 2023). In cancer settings, examining healthcare provider communication, the term 'therapeutic humility' emerged to describe a multi-component process consisting of 'relinquishing the need to "fix" along with tolerating ambiguity, accepting and honouring the patient as an expert, and trusting in the process' (Chochinov, 2023, p. 2884; Chochinov et al., 2013).

Humility is often associated with good communication skills, both verbal and non-verbal, and it sometimes emerges as a value in compassion-related writing in the medical literature (e.g., Fernando et al., 2016). As well as patients thinking that humility goes toward making a good (and by implication, compassionate) doctor (Nelson & Phi Huynh, 2023; Ruberton et al., 2016; Schnelle & Jones, 2023), so increasingly do doctors themselves (Chou et al., 2014; Mahant et al., 2012; Reynolds et al., 2023; Schnelle & Jones, 2022; Swendiman et al., 2019). In particular, one study identified humility as helpful in avoiding condescension to patients, and humility was thought to be more likely when doctors were confident in their own abilities, valued their patient's experiences and were open to the views of others (Wadhwa & Mahant, 2022).

Patient observers

It is the case that patients observe staff behaviour just as much as staff are involved in observing patients. Patients are easily able to discern the quality of the relationships between staff members and those with patients, and just as compassionate care and the expression of compassion are at least partly modelled and learnt in practice settings, patients have remarked that the same is true of care and contact that lacks compassion (Sinclair, McClement, et al., 2016).

Summary points

There are gaps in the literature about how different patient groups and different settings influence the expression and experience of compassion

The work of the nurse may be most frequently aligned with the emotional co-regulation of health-related shame

Patients can appreciate very brief, compassionate contact

Both common humanity and humility appear to be important in relation to compassion

Patients notice the quality of the relationships between members of the healthcare workforce that they see around them.

References

Baguley, S. I., Dev, V., Fernando, A. T., & Consedine, N. S. (2020). How do health professionals maintain compassion over time? Insights from a study of compassion in health. *Frontiers in Psychology, 11*(December), 1–11. https://doi.org/10.3389/fpsyg.2020.564554

Bivins, R., Tierney, S., & Seers, K. (2017). Compassionate care: Not easy, not free, not only nurses. *BMJ Quality and Safety, 26*(12), 1023–1026. https://doi.org/10.1136/bmjqs-2017-007005

Bond, C., Hui, A., Timmons, S., Wildbore, E., & Sinclair, S. (2022). Discourses of compassion from the margins of health care: The perspectives and experiences of people with a mental health condition. *Journal of Mental Health*. https://doi.org/10.1080/09638237.2022.2118692

Bramley, L., & Matiti, M. (2014). How does it really feel to be in my shoes? Patients' experiences of compassion within nursing care and their perceptions of developing compassionate nurses. *Journal of Clinical Nursing, 23*(19–20), 2790–2799. https://doi.org/10.1111/jocn.12537

Chochinov, H. M. (2023). Intensive caring: Reminding patients they matter. In *Journal of Clinical Oncology* (Vol. 41, Issue 16, pp. 2884–2887). Lippincott Williams and Wilkins. https://doi.org/10.1200/JCO.23.00042

Chochinov, H. M., McClement, S. E., Hack, T. F., McKeen, N. A., Rach, A. M., Gagnon, P., Sinclair, S., & Taylor-Brown, J. (2013). Health care provider communication: An empirical model of therapeutic effectiveness. *Cancer, 119*(9), 1706–1713. https://doi.org/10.1002/cncr.27949

Chou, C. M., Kellom, K., & Shea, J. A. (2014). Attitudes and habits of highly humanistic physicians. *Academic Medicine, 89*(9), 1252–1258. https://doi.org/10.1097/ACM.0000000000000405

Dev, V., Fernando, A. T., Kirby, J. N., & Consedine, N. S. (2019). Variation in the barriers to compassion across healthcare training and disciplines: A cross-sectional study of doctors, nurses, and medical students. *International Journal of Nursing Studies, 90*, 1–10. https://doi.org/10.1016/j.ijnurstu.2018.09.015

Durkin, J., Usher, K., & Jackson, D. (2019). Embodying compassion: A systematic review of the views of nurses and patients. *Journal of Clinical Nursing, 28*(9–10), 1380–1392. https://doi.org/10.1111/jocn.14722

Fernando, A. T., Arroll, B., & Consedine, N. S. (2016). Enhancing compassion in general practice: It's not all about the doctor. In *British Journal of General Practice* (Vol. 66, Issue 648, pp. 340–341). Royal College of General Practitioners. https://doi.org/10.3399/bjgp16X685741

Francis, R. (2013). Nursing. In *Volume 3. Report of the Mid Staffordshire NHS Foundation Trust Public Enquiry* (Vol. 3, pp. 1497–1539). The Stationery Office. https://www.gov.uk/government/publications/report-of-the-mid-staffordshire-nhs-foundation-trust-public-inquiry

Gillespie, A., & Reader, T. W. (2021). Identifying and encouraging high-quality healthcare: An analysis of the content and aims of patient letters of compliment. *BMJ Quality & Safety, 30*(6), 484–492. https://doi.org/10.1136/bmjqs-2019-010077

Goodrich, J. (2016). What makes a compassionate relationship between caregiver and patient ? Findings from the 'anniversary' Schwartz Rounds. *Journal of Compassionate Health Care*, 1–8. https://doi.org/10.1186/s40639-016-0026-7

Holmes, D. (2013). Mid Staffordshire scandal highlights NHS cultural crisis. *The Lancet, 381*(9866), 521–522. https://doi.org/10.1016/S0140-6736(13)60264-0

Jazaieri, H., Jinpa, G. T., McGonigal, K., Rosenberg, E. L., Finkelstein, J., Simon-Thomas, E., Cullen, M., Doty, J. R., Gross, J. J., & Goldin, P. R. (2013). Enhancing compassion: A randomized controlled trial of a compassion cultivation training program. *Journal of Happiness Studies, 14*(4), 1113–1126. https://doi.org/10.1007/s10902-012-9373-z

Kelly, M. A., Nixon, L., McClurg, C., Scherpbier, A., King, N., & Dornan, T. (2018). Experience of touch in health care: A meta-ethnography across the health care professions. *Qualitative Health Research, 28*(2), 200–212. https://doi.org/10.1177/1049732317707726

Lown, B. A., Rosen, J., & Marttila, J. (2011). An agenda for improving compassionate care: A survey shows about half of patients say such care is missing. *Health Affairs, 30*(9), 1772–1778. https://doi.org/10.1377/hlthaff.2011.0539

Mahant, S., Jovcevska, V., & Wadhwa, A. (2012). The nature of excellent clinicians at an academic health science center: A qualitative study. *Academic Medicine, 87*(12), 1715–1721. https://doi.org/10.1097/ACM.0b013e3182716790

Malenfant, S., Jaggi, P., Hayden, K. A., & Sinclair, S. (2022). Compassion in healthcare: An updated scoping review of the literature. *BMC Palliative Care, 21*(1), 1–28. https://doi.org/10.1186/s12904-022-00942-3

Menzies, E. P. (1960). A case study in the functioning of social systems as a defence against anxiety. A report on a study of the nursing service of a general hospital. *Human Relations, 13*, 95–121.

Nelson, C., & Phi Huynh, H. (2023). What do humble (and non-humble) doctors do? A mixed-method analysis of solicited patients' online reviews of humble and non-humble clinicians. In *North American Journal of Psychology* (Vol. 25, Issue 2).

Nettleton, S. (1995). The sociology of lay-professional interactions. In *The Sociology of Health and Illness* (First edition, pp. 131–159). Polity Press.

Nursing and Midwifery Council. (2018). *The Code. Professional standards of practice and behaviour for nurses, midwives and nursing associates.* www.nmc.org.uk/code

Patel, S., Pelletier-Bui, A., Smith, S., Roberts, M. B., Kilgannon, H., Trzeciak, S., & Roberts, B. W. (2019). Curricula for empathy and compassion training in medical education: A systematic review. *PLoS ONE, 14*(8), 1–25. https://doi.org/10.1371/journal.pone.0221412

Perry, B. (2008). Why exemplary oncology nurses seem to avoid compassion fatigue. *Canadian Oncology Nursing Journal = Revue Canadienne de Nursing Oncologique, 18*(2), 87–99. https://doi.org/10.5737/1181912x1828792

Perry, B. (2009). Conveying compassion through attention to the essential ordinary. *Nursing Older People, 21*(6), 1421.

Reynolds, C. W., Shen, M. R., Englesbe, M. J., & Kwakye, G. (2023). Humility: A revised definition and techniques for integration into surgical education. *Journal of the American College of Surgeons, 236*(6), 1261–1264. https://doi.org/10.1097/XCS.0000000000000640

Ruberton, P. M., Huynh, H. P., Miller, T. A., Kruse, E., Chancellor, J., & Lyubomirsky, S. (2016). The relationship between physician humility, physician–patient communication, and patient health. *Patient Education and Counseling, 99*(7), 1138–1145. https://doi.org/10.1016/j.pec.2016.01.012

Schnelle, C., & Jones, M. A. (2022). Qualitative study of medical doctors on their experiences and opinions of the characteristics of exceptionally good doctors. *Advances in Medical Education and Practice, 13*, 717–731. https://doi.org/10.2147/AMEP.S370980

Schnelle, C., & Jones, M. A. (2023). Characteristics of exceptionally good Doctors—A survey of public adults. *Heliyon, 9*(2). https://doi.org/10.1016/j.heliyon.2023.e13115

Schwartz, K. B. (1995, July 16). A patient's story. *The Boston Globe Magazine.* https://www.pointofcarefoundation.org.uk/our-work/schwartz-rounds/

Selman, L. E., Brighton, L. J., Sinclair, S., Karvinen, I., Egan, R., Speck, P., Powell, R. A., Deskur-Smielecka, E., Glajchen, M., Adler, S., Puchalski, C., Hunter, J., Gikaara, N., & Hope, J. (2018). Patients' and caregivers' needs, experiences, preferences and research priorities in spiritual care: A focus group study across nine countries. *Palliative Medicine, 32*(1), 216–230. https://doi.org/10.1177/0269216317734954

Sinclair, S., Beamer, K., Hack, T. F., McClement, S., Raffin Bouchal, S., Chochinov, H. M., & Hagen, N. A. (2017). Sympathy, empathy, and compassion: A grounded theory study of palliative care patients' understandings, experiences, and preferences. *Palliative Medicine, 31*(5), 437–447. https://doi.org/10.1177/0269216316663499

Sinclair, S., McClement, S., Raffin-Bouchal, S., Hack, T. F., Hagen, N. A., McConnell, S., & Chochinov, H. M. (2016). Compassion in health care: An empirical model. *Journal of Pain and Symptom Management, 51*(2), 193–203. https://doi.org/10.1016/j.jpainsymman.2015.10.009

Sinclair, S., Torres, M. B., Raffin-Bouchal, S., Hack, T. F., McClement, S., Hagen, N. A., & Chochinov, H. M. (2016). Compassion training in healthcare: What are patients' perspectives on training healthcare providers? *BMC Medical Education, 16*(1). https://doi.org/10.1186/s12909-016-0695-0

Singh, P., King-Shier, K., & Sinclair, S. (2018). The colours and contours of compassion: A systematic review of the perspectives of compassion among ethnically diverse patients and healthcare providers. In *PLoS ONE* (Vol. 13, Issue 5). Public Library of Science. https://doi.org/10.1371/journal.pone.0197261

Strauss, C., Lever Taylor, B., Gu, J., Kuyken, W., Baer, R., Jones, F., & Cavanagh, K. (2016). What is compassion and how can we measure it? A review of definitions and measures. *Clinical Psychology Review, 47*, 15–27. https://doi.org/10.1016/j.cpr.2016.05.004

Swendiman, R. A., Marcaccio, C. L., Han, J., Hoffman, D. I., Weiner, T. M., Nance, M. L., & Chou, C. M. (2019). Attitudes and habits of highly humanistic surgeons: A single-institution, mixed-methods study. *Academic Medicine, 94*(7), 1027–1032. https://doi.org/10.1097/ACM.0000000000002690

Thienprayoon, R., Sinclair, S., Lown, B. A., Pestian, T., Awtrey, E., Winick, N., & Kanov, J. (2022). Organizational compassion: Ameliorating healthcare worker's suffering and burnout. *Journal of Wellness, 4*(1), 3–5. https://doi.org/10.55504/2578-9333.1122

Tierney, S., Bivins, R., & Seers, K. (2019). Compassion in nursing: Solution or stereotype? *Nursing Inquiry, 26*(1). https://doi.org/10.1111/nin.12271

Tierney, S., Seers, K., Tutton, E., & Reeve, J. (2017). Enabling the flow of compassionate care: A grounded theory study. *BMC Health Services Research, 17*(1). https://doi.org/10.1186/s12913-017-2120-8

Trzeciak, S., & Mazzarelli, A. (2019a). *Compassionomics* (First edition). Studer group.

Trzeciak, S., & Mazzarelli, A. (2019b). The power of 40 seconds. In *Compassionomics. The Revolutionary Scientific Evidence that Caring Makes a Difference* (First edition, pp. 249–262). Studer Group, Llc.

Wadhwa, A., & Mahant, S. (2022). Humility in medical practice: A qualitative study of peer-nominated excellent clinicians. *BMC Medical Education, 22*(1). https://doi.org/10.1186/s12909-022-03146-8

Way, D., & Tracy, S. J. (2012). Conceptualizing compassion as recognizing, relating and (re)acting: A qualitative study of compassionate communication at hospice. *Communication Monographs, 79*(3), 292–315. https://doi.org/10.1080/03637751.2012.697630

Younas, A., Porr, C., Maddigan, J., Moore, J., Navarro, P., & Whitehead, D. (2023). Behavioural indicators of compassionate nursing care of individuals with complex needs: A naturalistic inquiry. *Journal of Clinical Nursing, 32*(13–14), 4024–4036. https://doi.org/10.1111/jocn.16542

7 Active engagement for compassion

This chapter presents the basic cognitive therapy model (CT model) and introduces mindfulness. The model for parsing out the four components of experience, used in combination with mindfulness, provides a powerful means of supporting compassionate action in healthcare. This skill set can increase the capacity to care for oneself whilst responding with sensitivity to the needs of others. It also helps to enhance personal and professional satisfaction when enacting compassion both routinely and when it is more difficult.

The cognitive therapy model

The CT model (Padesky & Mooney, 1990) expands on the work of Beck (1995) and is a framework that can be used to 'unpack' the four synergistic dimensions of human experience, namely physical sensations (biology), thoughts, emotions and behaviours, in response to any given situation or context. The model (see Figure 7.1) shows the links between the four dimensions and the capacity for each to both influence and be influenced by the other three.

There is a 'congruency' or 'match' between the four dimensions at any time. So, for example, if there is a joyful mood, the accompanying thoughts will be uplifting in nature, the body may feel light and energised, and impulses to act could include making arrangements to see friends or taking part in physical exercise. If there is a low mood, the accompanying thoughts will be somewhat gloomy, and the body may feel sluggish and slow. Associated behaviours for someone in this state might be less sociable and active and include avoiding contact with others or not taking exercise.

Biology, physiological state and physical sensations

Physical sensations arise from an underlying physiological state. They are experienced within and through the body and are influenced by

DOI: 10.4324/9781003427247-7

thoughts, emotions or actions that exert an influence on underlying physiological processes. Physical sensations can be slow to arise, for example, the onset of a tension headache, or appear very rapidly, like an increase in heartrate in response to an unpleasant shock when the threat processing system is activated. It is also the case that many physical sensations escape attention on a day-to-day basis. It is in this domain that stimulation of the oxytocin-opiate-parasympathetic system can be experienced as bodily feelings of safety, presence and connection.

Thoughts

Thoughts, visual images in the mind, memories of the past and daydreams about the future are all included in the 'cognitive' or thought component of the CT model. Interactions with others and responses to the ongoing context or environment are shaped by thoughts that interpret or give meaning to either internal (bodily) or external events. Speech, including both the words chosen and the tone of voice used, is the behavioural expression of thought. Compelling thoughts sometimes drive rapid and unwise actions in the heat of challenging situations, for example, in the middle of an argument, or can contribute significantly to a feeling of depletion and it is neither possible nor desirable to 'control' thinking. It is possible with mindfulness, however, to use the 'noticing' capacity of mind to recognise that unhelpful thinking is happening, to take a momentary pause and to choose what to say or do next on the basis of alternative thoughts that may encourage a more skilful relationship with any ongoing difficulties.

Emotions

Just as with thoughts, it is neither possible nor desirable to control emotions or moods and simply not possible to reliably evoke happiness or contentment, or to dispel anxiety at will. Unfortunately, sometimes this is seen as a personal failing and can lead to self-blame, but it is simply in the nature of emotions and a universal experience. As with thoughts, however, with mindfulness it is possible to become aware of an ongoing powerful emotional state, to take a momentary pause and to make skilful choices around how best to respond to it or relate to it.

Behaviour

Behaviour, actions, impulses and urges to act are the dimensions of experience where, provided the conditions for safety are met, there is the most freedom to choose a course of action. If there is a sufficient

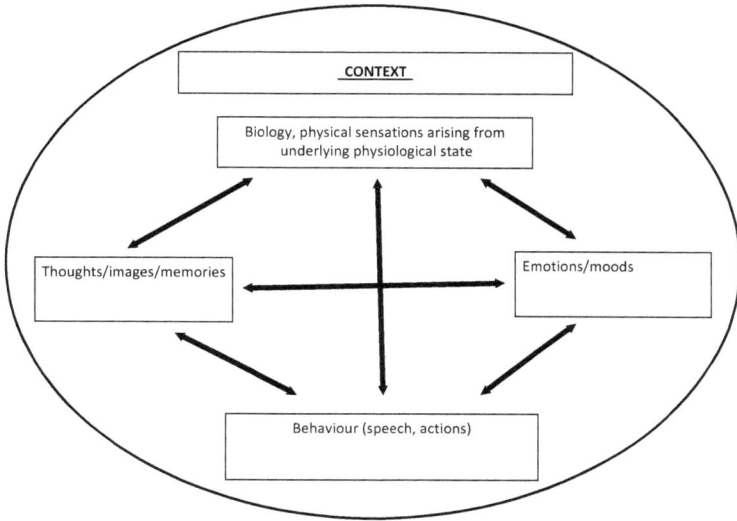

Figure 7.1 The Cognitive Therapy model. Adapted with permission of Christine A Padesky, PhD. © 1986 Center for Cognitive Therapy, Newport Beach, CA).

degree of mindful self-awareness to notice impulsivity or patterns of habitual responding, there is an opportunity to pause and decide what is most skilful to do or to avoid doing in that moment. Compassion is action-based and so expressed as a quality of behaviour.

Focus box 7.1   The Cognitive Therapy Model

Provides a method of parsing out experience into physical sensations, thoughts, emotions and behaviour in any context
Provides a helpful framework for understanding the dimensions of one's own reactions and the relationships between them
Provides a good foundation for using and understanding mindfulness

---

Mindfulness

Mindfulness meditation is a way of cultivating self-awareness (Tang et al., 2015) and of increasing the capacity for emotional self-regulation (Dorjee, 2016). Emotional regulation and more active self-care skills for the healthcare workforce have been identified as important in enhancing compassionate care in healthcare settings (Chochinov et al., 2013; Dev et al., 2019; Lown, 2016; Sinclair et al., 2023), and mindfulness provides the possibility of taking care of oneself whilst providing care and compassion to others in need. Mindfulness can also contribute to attentional awareness and the enjoyment of a compassionate practice, as well as supporting other dimensions of the 'four pillars of wellbeing', each of which are trainable ways of relating to oneself, other people and the experience of life, for flourishing and wellbeing (Dahl et al., 2020).

What is mindfulness?

Mindfulness involves deliberately paying attention to each moment as it unfolds. This process includes being open to one's own responses and holding them with kindness, curiosity and care, whilst cultivating a wise discernment to guide action, rather than being driven by thoughtless, impulsive or habitual reactivity (Kabat-Zinn, 2004). The nature of what is revealed, including reactions of aversion to those things that are unpleasant or difficult to bear, is held with sensitivity and self-compassion, since this illuminating attention only reveals what it is to be human and not a cause for blame. In this way, the capacity for an inclusive, whole hearted and more 'conscious living' is nurtured (Kabat-Zinn, 2004, p. 6). Using the four categories of experience as outlined in the CT model can help to bring further clarity to and understanding of one's own reactions to events and experiences and so contribute to social and emotional learning as a skill for self-care as well as professional expertise.

Learning mindfulness

Mindfulness, like compassion, is a reflexive and relational practice, and whilst the two are sometimes taught somewhat separately, mindfulness itself is imbued with compassion. Mindfulness is developed with the use of meditation as a form of brain training, and it gradually builds as a quality of mind and heart that is cultivated with patience and persistence, rather than with any forceful striving or strenuous effort.

When learning meditation, the breath and other sense-mediated experiences are used to 'anchor' the attention of the mind in the present moment; this is because the body, breath, sights, tastes and sounds are always present moment experiences. It is not possible to locate any bodily experience anywhere other than in the present moment; the body or breath of last week no longer exists, and the breath or body of next month has not yet come to fruition.

Physical sensations, including the breath entering and leaving the body, fluctuate sufficiently to capture the attention of the mind for long enough to begin to develop some degree of steady focus. It is a shared experience to have a mind that wanders, and whilst individual narratives differ, the process of mind wandering is a universal truth that invites patience and kindness. Physical sensations as present moment experiences are always available as anchors when the mind begins to travel back to old stories or spin fantasies about an existence somewhere in the future, and the raw sensory quality of sound, including that of speech, can also be also used as an anchor for practice as training progresses.

Mindfulness as emotion regulation

Buddhist psychology teaches that when thoughts, emotions and physical feelings or a particular turn of events are experienced as pleasant or welcome, the reaction is to want to prolong or repeat them. If experiences are unpleasant, the human reaction is to want to push them away or to engage in a usually futile struggle to make things different in order to avoid personal distress. Some experiences register as neither pleasant nor unpleasant and can provoke feelings of boredom or of being under-stimulated.

Each of these responses is entirely normal and 'perfectly human' and often go unnoticed unless events are very clearly pleasant or unpleasant. Subtle efforts to perpetuate the pleasant and to avoid the unpleasant, however, can become problematic for healthcare professionals, as it is in the nature of their work to repeatedly encounter suffering that provokes an empathic response involving unpleasant feelings. Sometimes this results in healthcare worker distress when it is felt that the suffering is too much and this can reduce the capacity of the healthcare worker to provide compassionate care to others.

Mindfulness teaches that whilst we have little control over what happens in life, it is possible to learn to respond skilfully and with equanimity to the challenges when they arise, rather than to react in ways that are thoughtless and habitual. Whilst mindfulness in its fullest sense is a distinct and ethically informed way of relating to oneself and others in the world and not just a series of strategies, a modest mindfulness practice can strengthen emotional self-regulation skills effectively and help to cultivate steadiness and patience. Furthermore, it is useful to have the experience of being engaged in a conscious practice of emotional self-regulation for oneself as a portal into the experience of intentionally co-regulating the emotions of others as part of a skilled, compassionate practice.

Unskilful reactivity, expressed as words and actions, can cause harm of different sorts to others as well as to oneself. If there is anger or irritation, important relationships may be fractured or damaged and difficult to repair thereafter, and if there is overwhelm and distress, action can be taken without due consideration and become a source of regret at a later date. Furthermore, it is a common experience that unskilful reactions are often followed by protracted periods of time when the threat processing system continues to be active because of a ruminative mind that is unable to 'let go' and move on, long beyond the point at which any post-event reflection has been useful.

Focus box 7.2   Human reactions to experience

To want to prolong or repeat pleasant experiences,
To want to terminate or avoid unpleasant experiences
To be uninterested in what is neither pleasant nor unpleasant

---

Fusing, identifying and acting from within reactive mind and body states

A mindful awareness allows thoughts, emotions and physical sensations, all of which can be powerful drivers of behaviour, to be seen clearly and known for what they are. Mindfulness offers a way of 'stepping out of' a stream of turbulent thoughts, strong emotions and impulses to act rashly that can be overwhelming. The approach does not involve fixing emotions, or controlling thoughts, or trying to eliminate the unpleasant but instead learning to relate to the momentum and emotional charge of the moment in a more flexible way. The aim of mindfulness is to stay 'in touch' with the difficulty, to understand that there may be some degree of activation of the threat processing system, but not to be overwhelmed by it, or to act from within it. As a result, there is an increased sense of perspective, agency and choice.

Mindfulness can offer practical ways of dealing with difficult situations. For example, feeling in to the physical sense of the height and weight and shape of one's own body helps to ground and stabilise in the moment and facilitates a steady attunement to the patient whilst reducing the likelihood of emotional contagion and overwhelm if strong emotions are running high, in either oneself or the patient.

Mindfulness also teaches practical steps towards cultivating a kinder and wiser self to 'accompany' oneself in difficult times. This is a noticing and observing self that no longer 'fuses' or 'identifies' so easily with unwanted mood and mind states, but one that is able to recognise what is happening and stay balanced and centred, nonetheless. Any impulsivity generated by a reactive mind and body state is observed by a gentle and kind self that remains connected with professional values and the intention to remain compassionate to oneself and to others. Reactive mind and body states are acknowledged, but they do not 'run the show'.

When there is a difficult interaction that is still 'alive' in the mind and body, if the threat processing system is still activated, this arousal can carry over to colour and shape the quality of the next encounter, whether that is with a colleague or a patient. A mindful pause can be used to disengage from reactive thinking, to gain perspective and to re-centre before carrying on. Possibility and flexible thinking begin to open up in a more expansive mind, previously one contracted around the preoccupations of any ongoing difficulty. A brief pause can also be used to interrupt any unhelpful internal momentum that may be gaining traction in a difficult encounter with a patient or colleague in much the same way.

Enjoying compassion

Mindfulness helps to reduce the negative effects of the 'push and pull' experiences of life that fragment thinking and disperse the capacity for care and attention. It helps a faster settling of the threat processing system back to 'base line' once immediate difficulties have passed or resolved (Crosswell et al., 2017), and the increased capacity for attention can also be deployed to noticing small moments of compassionate or joyful contact with patients or colleagues that also play a part in supporting wellbeing.

Attunement

The flexibility of attention learnt in mindfulness allows the intentional and skilful division of attention between oneself and the needs of another person. The quality of the attention that is afforded to another person in an encounter is also instrumental in generating feelings of presence and connection (Jha, 2020), key features of the experience of compassion as reported by patients. Mindfulness illuminates the flow of internal thoughts, emotions, physical sensations and impulses to act in oneself that are both influencing and are influenced by the bio-behavioural signals of another person. A conscious awareness of an interaction with another person, as it unfolds also allows space in which to refresh the intention to act with compassion, an intention that is in alignment with professional values and supports skilful action and personal and professional satisfaction.

Mindfulness, compassion and the professional commitment to care

Processes of categorising people as members of 'in' or 'out' groups are automatic and unconscious (Fiske, 2008) and can skew perceptions of other people in fundamental ways (e.g., Woitzel et al., 2024).

A combination of the CT model and mindfulness can be used 'live' and 'in the moment' to care for and attend to precisely these and other difficulties that may be faced by healthcare professionals, and so to support the intention to be 'healing and not harmful'. The model can also be used for after-event reflection and learning for oneself and others when opportunities arise. Contextual factors, including any organisational shortcomings, safety and personal experience, may all be included and considered as barriers and facilitators of compassion, as they were present in that situation.

Leaders in the field of mindfulness and social justice are exploring the power of mindfulness to heal experiences of racism and encouraging those inhabiting white racialised bodies to develop a mindful awareness of their own identity-based biases (King, 2018; Magee, 2019). It is known that a mindful sensitivity to one's own automatic responses enables unhelpful reactions based on any form of 'othering' to come into awareness more quickly than without (Chang et al., 2023). Once revealed, the use of mindfulness is a first step towards detoxifying processes of harmful othering and replacing them with a more inclusive approach to compassion that is aligned with professional values.

Focus box 7.3   Benefits of mindfulness for healthcare professionals

Helps to take care of oneself 'in the moment' with emotional regulation strategies
Increased attunement to the needs of other people
Reduces the likelihood of unskilful automaticity and reactivity
Helps to remain steady and grounded in difficult situations

Mindfulness research

High quality evidence supporting the personal benefits of mindfulness training for healthcare professionals continues to accrue (Kajee et al., 2024). Developing a mindfulness practice can help concentration over periods of intensive demand, such as that seen in healthcare settings (Jha et al., 2017), and there is good evidence that mindfulness helps to reduce habitual emotional reactivity in favour of appropriate and thoughtful responding under conditions of challenge and pressure (Quaglia et al., 2019).

The process of decentring (the process of obtaining distance from, or getting a different perspective on, something) from intensity during decision making, is also associated with a healthier physiological state

(Grossmann et al., 2016), and decentring itself is thought to be a key process in the benefits conferred by mindfulness training courses (Hanley et al., 2021). More specifically, the acquisition of mindfulness skills is thought to be an essential step that should be included when devising compassion education for healthcare professionals (Sinclair et al., 2023).

Summary points

Mindfulness helps with emotional regulation

Mindfulness helps appreciate one's own professionalism and good intentions

Mindfulness helps appreciate moments of joyful connection with others to nourish and replenish the capacity for compassion

Mindfulness supports making skilful and compassionate choices for oneself and others in key moments

References

Beck, J. S. (1995). Cognitive conceptualisation. In *Cognitive Therapy. Basics and Beyond* (First edition, pp. 13–24). The Guildford Press.

Chang, D. F., Donald, J., Whitney, J., Miao, I. Y., & Sahdra, B. (2023). Does mindfulness improve intergroup bias, internalized bias, and anti-bias outcomes?: A meta-analysis of the evidence and agenda for future research. *Personality and Social Psychology Bulletin.* https://doi.org/10.1177/01461672231178518

Chochinov, H. M., McClement, S. E., Hack, T. F., McKeen, N. A., Rach, A. M., Gagnon, P., Sinclair, S., & Taylor-Brown, J. (2013). Health care provider communication: An empirical model of therapeutic effectiveness. *Cancer, 119*(9), 1706–1713. https://doi.org/10.1002/cncr.27949

Crosswell, A. D., Moreno, P. I., Raposa, E. B., Motivala, S. J., Stanton, A. L., Ganz, P. A., & Bower, J. E. (2017). Effects of mindfulness training on emotional and physiologic recovery from induced negative affect. *Psychoneuroendocrinology, 86,* 78–86. https://doi.org/10.1016/j.psyneuen.2017.08.003

Dahl, C. J., Wilson-Mendenhall, C. D., & Davidson, R. J. (2020). The plasticity of well-being: A training-based framework for the cultivation of human flourishing. *Proceedings of the National Academy of Sciences of the United States of America, 117*(51), 32197–32206. https://doi.org/10.1073/pnas.2014859117

Dev, V., Fernando, A. T., Kirby, J. N., & Consedine, N. S. (2019). Variation in the barriers to compassion across healthcare training and disciplines: A cross-sectional study of doctors, nurses, and medical students. *International Journal of Nursing Studies, 90,* 1–10. https://doi.org/10.1016/j.ijnurstu.2018.09.015

Dorjee, D. (2016). Defining contemplative science: The metacognitive self-regulatory capacity of the mind, context of meditation practice and modes of existential awareness. *Frontiers in Psychology, 7*(November), 1–15. https://doi.org/10.3389/fpsyg.2016.01788

Fiske, S. T. (2008). *Look twice.* https://greatergood.berkeley.edu/article/item/look_twice

Grossmann, I., Sahdra, B. K., & Ciarrochi, J. (2016). A heart and a mind: Self-distancing facilitates the association between heart rate variability, and wise reasoning. *Frontiers in Behavioral Neuroscience, 10*(April), 1–10. https://doi.org/10.3389/fnbeh.2016.00068

Hanley, A. W., de Vibe, M., Solhaug, I., Farb, N., Goldin, P. R., Gross, J. J., & Garland, E. L. (2021). Modeling the mindfulness-to-meaning theory's mindful reappraisal hypothesis: Replication with longitudinal data from a randomized controlled study. *Stress and Health, 37*(4), 778–789. https://doi.org/10.1002/smi.3035

Jha, A. P. (2020). *The brain science of attention and overwhelm.* Www.Mindful.Org. https://www.mindful.org/youre-overwhelmed-and-its-not-your-fault/

Jha, A. P., Witkin, J. E., Morrison, A. B., Rostrup, N., & Stanley, E. (2017). Short-form mindfulness training protects against working memory degradation over high-demand intervals. *Journal of Cognitive Enhancement, 1*(2), 154–171. https://doi.org/10.1007/s41465-017-0035-2

Kabat-Zinn, J. (2004). What is mindfulness? In *Wherever You Go, There You Are. Mindfulness Meditation for Everyday Life* (Retitled edition, pp. 3–7). Piatkus.

Kajee, N., Montero-Marin, J., Saunders, K. E. A., Myall, K., Harriss, E., & Kuyken, W. (2024). Mindfulness training in healthcare professions: A scoping review of systematic reviews. In *Medical Education.* John Wiley and Sons Inc. https://doi.org/10.1111/medu.15293

King, R. (2018). *Mindful of Race* (First edition). Sounds True.

Lown, B. A. (2016). A social neuroscience-informed model for teaching and practising compassion in health care. *Medical Education, 50*(3), 332–342. https://doi.org/10.1111/medu.12926

Magee, R. V. (2019). *The Inner Work of Racial Justice* (First edition). Tarcher Perigree.

Mendoza-Denton, R. (2016, July 27). *How to stop the racist in you.* https://greatergood.berkeley.edu/article/item/how_to_stop_the_racist_in_you

Padesky, C. A., & Mooney, K. A. (1990). Presenting the cognitive model to clients. *International Cognitive Therapy Newsletter, 6*, 13–14. https://www.padesky.com/clinical-corner/publications/

Quaglia, J. T., Zeidan, F., Grossenbacher, P. G., Freeman, S. P., Braun, S. E., Martelli, A., Goodman, R. J., & Brown, K. W. (2019). Brief mindfulness training enhances cognitive control in socioemotional contexts: Behavioral and neural evidence. *PLoS ONE, 14*(7), 1–21. https://doi.org/10.1371/journal.pone.0219862

Sinclair, S., Harris, D., Kondejewski, J., Roze des Ordons, A. L., Jaggi, P., & Hack, T. F. (2023). Program leaders' and educators' perspectives on the factors impacting the implementation and sustainment of compassion training programs: A qualitative study, teaching and learning in medicine. *Teaching and Learning in Medicine, 35*(1), 21–36. https://doi.org/10.1080/10401334.2021.2017941

Tang, Y.-Y., Hölzel, B. K., & Posner, M. I. (2015). The neuroscience of mindfulness meditation. *Nature Reviews Neuroscience, 16*(5), 312–312. https://doi.org/10.1038/nrn3954

Woitzel, J., Ingendahl, M., & Alves, H. (2024). Intergroup bias in perceived trustworthiness among few or many minimal groups. *Journal of Experimental Social Psychology, 115.* https://doi.org/10.1016/j.jesp.2024.104668

8 Empathic concern and compassion

Professional practices

The capacity for compassion in humans was originally developed as a nuturing strategy in the context of close family groups, rather than as an expression of care offered to strangers, as it has become in contemporary health and social care settings. This chapter considers the particularities and similarities of empathic concern and compassion as professional practices within the context of healthcare. Ways of reliably connecting to the motivation or intention to be compassionate are discussed.

Empathic concern

Whilst the terms empathic concern (or empathy aimed at relieving suffering in patients) and compassion are sometimes used without distinction, here they are treated relatively separately to reflect both current compassion theory (e.g., Gilbert, 2020; Strauss et al., 2016) and neurophysiological evidence (Singer & Klimecki, 2014). These and other sources converge around two ideas: firstly, that the threat processing system comprising the amygdala, the pituitary-adrenal axis and the sympathetic nervous system is activated in the healthcare worker during the empathic response, and secondly, that this system is suppressed by the oxytocin-opiate-parasympathetic system as an integral part of the compassionate response itself. These two 'phases' therefore also involve entirely different emotional experiences and behavioural responses, and both are important in understanding what is demanded of the healthcare worker as part of a compassionate response. The empathic response is triggered on the initial exposure to suffering and is associated with unpleasant emotions and a tendency to withdraw from the source of suffering, whilst the compassionate response that follows is associated with approaching to help relieve suffering and pleasant emotions.

Empathic concern (Batson, 2017) is thought to be necessary for the recognition of suffering, however, and it is thought that a lack of empathic concern on the part of healthcare professionals may increase the risk of some groups of people being overlooked in relation to their health care

DOI: 10.4324/9781003427247-8

needs or, alternatively, exposed to care that lacks compassion, or both. Empathy, like compassion, is also a relational or interpersonal practice and is 'a continuous process of … attempting to understand another's distinct emotional perspective on matters of personal significance' (Main et al., 2017, p. 360). Therefore, in the context of healthcare, this necessarily involves obtaining the patient's views and preferences wherever possible in order to relieve suffering in the patient.

Focus box 8.1   Features of empathic concern (or empathy for patient benefit) in healthcare

Necessary for the recognition of suffering
Requires effective management of any unpleasant feelings on the part of the healthcare worker as they arise
Involves finding out what the patient wants
Involves using professional skills to plan effective action to relieve or prevent suffering

---

A shared humanity

Invoking the sense of a shared humanity with patients is already known to be used spontaneously by some healthcare workers to support a compassionate attitude over time (Baguley et al., 2020). This attitude may be inclusive of the understanding of a shared vulnerability to the vicissitudes of life, including those of of illness or ill health specifically, and also resonates with reports that the experience of personal illness in healthcare workers facilitates the expression of compassion towards their patients more easily (Roberts et al., 2011). An understanding of a shared humanity as applied to health and social care is also based on the notion that, in fundamental ways, the people seen in health and social care settings are not so very different from the people that care for them in those same settings. Reality also teaches that the boundaries between being a patient and a member of the healthcare workforce are fluid at best and can change rapidly and very dramatically.

Cultivating the *sense of a shared humanity with patients* or *the identification with all of humanity* (Condon & Makransky, 2020a, 2020b) can provide a channel for a caring connection with other unknown people and forms an important part of some compassion training programmes. It is also possible, however, to explore and cultivate this understanding outside of a formal training programme in order to widen the circle of care and concern beyond a narrow grouping of family and friends to other people who are in need of compassion. Cultivating the sense of a common humanity actively overcomes behaviour rooted in an evolutionary past that can result in the tendency to be reluctant to offer compassion to strangers when compared to offering compassion to people who are either close or familiar in some way.

The understanding of a shared humanity provides a sense of connection and healthy relatedness with other people at a fundamental level without necessarily needing to know the details of their lives, and a relatedness that may be less prone to distressing personalisation. It can increase the 'relevance' of the suffering of another person (Mascaro, 2024) and helps to reduce 'othering', unhelpful social comparisons and inadvertently contributing to identity-based harms, whilst allowing for the need to remain sensitive to the individual and their context.

There are also the understandings that all individuals have a deeply held wish to be happy and to avoid suffering (Jazaieri et al., 2013) and that each person has their own intrinsic worth, dignity and potential (Condon & Makransky, 2020a). It is not necessary to know a patient or a colleague well in order to gently remind oneself of the aspirations that they will have to be happy, to be free from suffering and to live with dignity and fulfil their potential, since those are wishes that everyone shares.

The understanding of a shared humanity as it is applied in Kristin Neff and Christopher Germer's self-compassion training courses is also useful in healthcare (e.g., Neff, 2011; Neff et al., 2020). Common humanity in their courses is considered a powerful vehicle for connection with other people because of an openness to, and embracing of, the fallibility and imperfection of human nature, and not in spite of it. This is another attitudinal understanding that may help to reduce unnecessary judgement and unhelpful distance from patients who are often seeking compassionate connection to ease states of health-related shame and fear.

Interconnectedness

Cultivating other understandings of the way that human beings are *deeply interconnected and reliant upon each other* may comprise another pathway to empathic concern or motivate compassionate action. This understanding can be developed by reflecting on a shared reliance on the actions of countless unknown others for the basic necessities of life, for example, the people who are involved in the production of food and medicines, run transport systems and take care of waste disposal. Health and social care facilities themselves are hubs of cooperation between different sets of people with varying roles involved in caring for others.

Much of this book also speaks to the nature of the evolved and embodied communication systems that are mutually influencing and seek connection. 'We are not made for exclusivity or self-sufficiency but for interdependence. We break this law of our being at our own peril …

it is as simple and difficult as that.' (Tutu & Tutu, 2014, p. 215). To recall the reliance on others that is shared by all human beings goes to the heart of what it is to be human and is another shared commonality between healthcare professionals and their patients.

Self-identity and compassion

Reconnecting with the *professional aspiration to be of benefit to others* may also offer a further pathway to compassionate intention because many of the people in healthcare have chosen a self and professional identity that is associated with compassion. It is also the case that some healthcare workers are motivated to a state of empathic concern by personal beliefs and experiences in ways that nourish and do not deplete or distress them. These are other pathways that can be appropriately enacted within the boundaries of professional relationships with patients.

Focus box 8.2   Notions of common humanity/ interconnectedness or a professional aspiration to be compassionate can overcome preference on the basis of

Family
Friendship
Familiarity of some sort

Compassion

Compassion is realised through action or behaviour (Feldman, 2017). Compassionate care consists of a blend of profession-specific competencies or role-related proficiencies and relational skills for the emotional co-regulation of states of health-related fear and shame. These skills are practised in response to the needs of the patient, in the moment, as they arise, and part of what it means to practise compassion skilfully is to be attuned to the patient and sensitive to any opportunities to offer compassion when they emerge. Tuning in to changes in the flow of ease or tension in the quality of the contact provides a means of immediate feedback that helps to gauge what is required in the next moment as the situation unfolds. The felt changes and shifts in the flow within the interaction are reflective of stimulation or activity in the two opposing neurophysiological systems. One relating to threat processing and the other, the care-giving and compassion system, and both are responsive to the emotionally co-regulating effect of bio-behavioural signalling that is implicit in verbal and non-verbal communication.

The capacity to respond flexibly and with compassion can be enhanced on the basis of the supporting factors available to each individual in that moment, and each represents another variation in the professional work of compassion in health and social care settings. Either drawing upon the identification of a shared humanity, 'feeling in to' the sense of oneself as a compassionate person or professional, or holding close to the intention to be compassionate, or more likely, a blend of these different supporting factors, are all skilful ways of relating to people in need.

The intention to remain compassionate can be renewed in each moment as an ongoing commitment to patient care. Mindfulness strategies can be used to allow any difficulties to be held in awareness whilst making skilful choices that are in alignment with personal and professional values and supportive of one's own wellbeing. It is also possible for healthcare professionals to use mindfulness to acknowledge and appreciate the skilful nature of their own compassionate intentions and actions in the face of difficulty and in situations that are challenging.

Sometimes healthcare workers overlook opportunities to practice compassion (Patel et al., 2019), but healthcare professionals may also under-value the degree to which momentary expressions of compassionate contact and compassionate care are appreciated and experienced as meaningful by patients (e.g., Schwartz, 1995; What your patient is thinking, 2023). These tiny havens of human connection can be held in awareness, either briefly in the moment or as part of an intentional practice at a later time, and can help to increase enjoyment and contribute to healthier mental and physical states (Rick Hanson, 2009) in the healthcare workforce. Offering or expressing compassion is always person-centred and responsive to the need of the patient in that moment. The professional practice of compassion is, however, also inclusive of and balanced with the health and needs of oneself, along with any professional obligations and responsibilities that are present.

Focus box 8.3   Characteristics of compassion in healthcare

Expressed through behaviour (blends of emotional co-regulation skills + other profession-specific competencies)
Patient-centred
Moment-specific
Context-sensitive
Inclusive of the needs of oneself

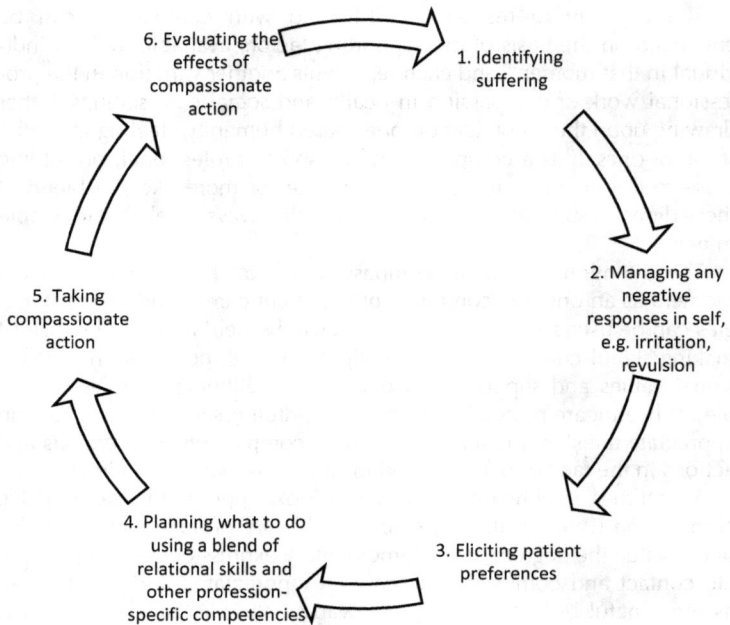

Figure 8.1 Empathic concern and compassion as an iterative process.

Whilst empathic concern and compassion activate distinct neural circuitry and are emotionally very different entities (Ricard, 2015), in practice, they are closely related processes and can blend together to form an iterative process designed to relieve suffering. The process begins with the identification of suffering (empathic concern) and concludes with evaluating the effects of compassionate action, that is, compassion itself, in order to establish if there is further suffering to be relieved (see Figure 8.1).

Compassion and role

Opportunities for practising compassion and the barriers encountered are known to vary by discipline and level of seniority or training for nurses and doctors, almost certainly because of their different role responsibilities (Dev et al., 2019). Other healthcare personnel, across a range of different health and social care systems and services, will also have, as a result of their role, greater, fewer, or different, opportunities to practise and refine emotional co-regulation skills for health-related fear and shame as part of compassionate care.

Humility and compassion

Humility relates to the capacity of the healthcare worker to become involved in the effective emotional co-regulation of the patient experience of shame, in particular. From a patient perspective, humility on the part of the healthcare worker is associated with a helpful presence, and a lack of humility has been found to be associated with shame and feeling dismissed (Nelson & Phi Huynh, 2023). Humility in healthcare more generally has been interpreted as knowing one's limits and appreciating the role of others, including that of the patient (Cauble et al., 2022; Michalec, 2023), and it has been pointed out that humility within a relationship does not remove any professionalism, self-respect or personal satisfaction involved in doing a job well and celebrates rather than opposes excellence (Spezio et al., 2019).

Humility has been described as a position of balance between an inflated sense of self-importance and a devaluation of one's worth (Smith & Bellitto, 2023), and is thought to have both a personal component that includes self-compassion and a relational component that regards other people as just as valuable or worthy as oneself (Chancellor & Lyubomirsky, 2013). Whilst humility is attitudinal and can be developed or increased in response to new experiences and changes in perspective, as with compassion itself, it is expressed through behaviour. Contemplating and reflecting on the intrinsic worth, potential and dignity of all people (Condon & Makransky, 2020b, 2020a), in combination with a sense of connection and inter-reliance of all human beings, can help to cultivate a greater sense of humility with accompanying changes in speech and other actions.

Humility has been described as a relational lubricant (Van Tongeren et al., 2019), and it also functions as a social surfactant. These two properties of humility combined, permit a healthy accommodation of the power differentials that are embedded within healthcare delivery itself (Michalec et al., 2024) and that are sometimes very large and difficult for patients to navigate within relationships with healthcare professionals (Nettleton, 1995).

Humility can change the nature of the contact between the healthcare worker and patient from one of relationship to that of partnership, where contributions to the partnership are different but equally valued, and compassion may be expressed and experienced more fully and without reservation. It is also a partnership that avoids vulnerable patients feeling shamed in the presence of a healthcare worker, who may be a 'socially more powerful player' in the encounter (DasGupta, 2008, p. 981) and experienced as overbearing as a result.

The nature of this partnership does not preclude the possession of specialist skills, sophisticated knowledge and responsibility on the part of members of the healthcare workforce. Instead, it points to the degree of care and attention that are required to contribute to a partnership in a way that ensures the threat processing system is not activated on the basis of shame or fear and conditions are conducive for the experience of compassion on the part of the patient. Mindfulness skills allow attunement to the ebb and flow of the interaction on the part of the healthcare worker who, whilst being aware of their own influence, can make skilled adjustments to the quality of their communication to ensure that the interaction is fulfilling the emotional co-regulatory function of compassion.

Focus box 8.4   Humility in relationships with patients

Can transform the patient-professional relationship to one of partnership

Is expressed through the quality of behaviour (speech + other behavioural vectors)

Is transmitted through bio-behavioural signalling implicit in communication

Avoids activation of the threat processing system by imbalances of power in the relationship and shame specifically

Facilitates the experience of compassion for patients

Compassion is defined by patients

Patients are able to tell from the visceral or felt-experience of connection or presence during an interaction with a healthcare worker if they have experienced compassion or not (see Chapter 6). On the occasions when compassion is experienced, there is a congruency between the needs of the patient and the quality of contact offered by the healthcare worker. When compassion is not experienced, it does not necessarily mean that the healthcare worker was not offering compassion, but instead, that what was offered did not or could not meet the needs of the patient, in some way, at that point in time. To the extent that it is possible, the sources of any mismatch between the expectations held by the patient and what was possible for the healthcare worker to offer can be explored to provide increased understanding and used as a learning opportunity.

The stewardship of compassion

The extent to which patients or the people who are close to them appear to be able to engage with and co-create relationships with healthcare professionals so that a caring and compassionate connection can be established will exist somewhere on a continuum. Patients themselves may move up and down on the continuum, consistent with increments of improvement or deterioration in their condition.

As a result of the effects of some illnesses, for example advanced dementia, the capacity for people to respond clearly or positively to compassionate bio-behavioural signalling may be impeded. People with very challenging behaviour may also be at particular risk of care that lacks compassion and sometimes constitutes cruelty and neglect. It is in these circumstances that the role of health and social care staff as the guardians of compassion is most critical.

The conscious and intentional use of compassionate means to bring comfort and effect emotional co-regulation obtained from offering human presence and connection to everyone seen in health and social care systems, but especially those known to be at risk, is essential work.

Compassion in health and social care is a collective responsibility, however, and all leaders in health and social care have a vital role in the stewardship of compassion as a valued quality of care. They are charged with ensuring that their organisations provide the conditions that are conducive for compassion to flourish and for taking remedial action when they are not.

Summary points

The capacity for compassion developed in the context of small family groups in an evolutionary past

Compassion is offered to unknown others as part of a professional practice in healthcare

Identifying with a shared humanity may make it easier to offer compassion to strangers

Identifying with a shared humanity can also find expression as humility of action

Connecting with professional aspirations may make it easier to offer compassion to strangers

Compassion in healthcare includes being competent in both relational skills for emotional co-regulation of fear and shame, and any other profession-specific skills necessary for the care of the patient

References

Baguley, S. I., Dev, V., Fernando, A. T., & Consedine, N. S. (2020). How do health professionals maintain compassion over time? Insights from a study of compassion in health. *Frontiers in Psychology, 11*(December), 1–11. https://doi.org/10.3389/fpsyg.2020.564554

Batson, C. D. (2017). The empathy-altruism hypothesis: What and so what? In E. M. Seppala, E. Simon-Thomas, S. L. Brown, M. C. Worline, D. C. Cameron, &

J. R. Doty (Eds.), *The Oxford Handbook of Compassion Science* (First edition, pp. 27–40). Oxford University Press.

Cauble, M. R., Said, I. A., McLaughlin, A. T., Gazaway, S., Van Tongeren, D. R., Hook, J. N., Lacey, E. K., Davis, E. B., & Davis, D. E. (2022). Religion/spirituality and the twin virtues of humility and gratitude. In *Handbook of Positive Psychology, Religion, and Spirituality* (pp. 379–393). Springer International Publishing. https://doi.org/10.1007/978-3-031-10274-5_24

Chancellor, J., & Lyubomirsky, S. (2013). Humble beginnings: Current trends, state perspectives, and hallmarks of humility. *Social and Personality Psychology Compass*, 7(11), 819–833. https://doi.org/10.1111/spc3.12069

Condon, P., & Makransky, J. (2020a). Recovering the relational starting point of compassion training: A foundation for sustainable and inclusive care. *Perspectives on Psychological Science*, 15(6), 1346–1362. https://doi.org/10.1177/1745691620922200

Condon, P., & Makransky, J. (2020b). Sustainable compassion training: Integrating meditation theory with psychological science. *Frontiers in Psychology*, 11. https://doi.org/10.3389/fpsyg.2020.02249

DasGupta, S. (2008). Narrative humility. In *Lancet* (Vol. 371, Issue 9617, pp. 980–981). https://doi.org/10.1016/S0140-6736(08)60440-7

Dev, V., Fernando, A. T., Kirby, J. N., & Consedine, N. S. (2019). Variation in the barriers to compassion across healthcare training and disciplines: A cross-sectional study of doctors, nurses, and medical students. *International Journal of Nursing Studies*, 90, 1–10. https://doi.org/10.1016/j.ijnurstu.2018.09.015

Feldman C. (2017). Compassion. In Boundless Heart. The Buddha's Path of Kindness, Compassion, Joy and Equanimity. (First edition). Shambhala.

Gilbert, P. (2020). Compassion: From its evolution to a psychotherapy. *Frontiers in Psychology*, 11(December). https://doi.org/10.3389/fpsyg.2020.586161

Jazaieri, H., Jinpa, G., McGonigal, K., Rosenberg, E. L., Finkelstein, J., Simon-Thomas, E., Cullen, M., Doty, J. R., Gross, J. J., & Goldin, P. R. (2013). Enhancing compassion: A randomized controlled trial of a compassion cultivation training program. *Journal of Happiness Studies*, 14(4), 1113–1126. https://doi.org/10.1007/s10902-012-9373-z

Main, A., Walle, E. A., Kho, C., & Halpern, J. (2017). The interpersonal functions of empathy: A relational perspective. *Emotion Review*, 9(4), 358–366. https://doi.org/10.1177/1754073916669440

Mascaro, J. (2024, August). *The Science of Compassion*. Mind and Life Institute. https://www.mindandlife.org/insight/the-science-of-compassion/

Michalec, B. (for additional references). (2023). *A researcher's prescription for better health care: A dose of humility for doctors, nurses and clinicians*. https://theconversation.com/a-researchers-prescription-for-better-health-care-a-dose-of-humility-for-doctors-nurses-and-clinicians-210175?utm_source=Receive+News+from+the+John+Templeton+Foundation&utm_campaign=afc5172588-EMAIL_CAMPAIGN_2023_possibilities_20231206&utm_medium=email&utm_term=0_-938f7e3a64-%5BLIST_EMAIL_ID%5D

Michalec, B., Cuddy, M. M., Felix, K., Gur-Arie, R., Tilburt, J. C., & Hafferty, F. W. (2024). Positioning humility within healthcare delivery - From doctors' and nurses' perspectives. *Human Factors in Healthcare*, 5. https://doi.org/10.1016/j.hfh.2023.100061

Neff, K. D. (2011). Self-compassion, self-esteem, and well-being. *Social and Personality Psychology Compass, 5*(1), 1–12. https://doi.org/10.1111/j.1751-9004.2010.00330.x

Neff, K. D., Knox, M. C., Long, P., & Gregory, K. (2020). Caring for others without losing yourself: An adaptation of the mindful self-compassion program for healthcare communities. *Journal of Clinical Psychology, 76*(9), 1543–1562. https://doi.org/10.1002/jclp.23007

Nelson, C., & Phi Huynh, H. (2023). What do humble (and non-humble) doctors do? A mixed-method analysis of solicited patients' online reviews of humble and non-humble clinicians. *North American Journal of Psychology, 25*(2).

Nettleton, S. (1995). The sociology of lay-professional interactions. In *The Sociology of Health and Illness* (First edition, pp. 131–159). Polity Press.

Patel, S., Pelletier-Bui, A., Smith, S., Roberts, M. B., Kilgannon, H., Trzeciak, S., & Roberts, B. W. (2019). Curricula for empathy and compassion training in medical education: A systematic review. *PLoS ONE, 14*(8), 1–25. https://doi.org/10.1371/journal.pone.0221412

Ricard, M. (2015). From empathy to compassion in a neuroscience laboratory. In *Altruism. The Power of Compassion to Change Yourself and the World* (pp. 56–64). Little, Brown and Company.

Rick Hanson. (2009, November 1). *Taking in the good.* https://greatergood.berkeley.edu/article/item/taking_in_the_good

Roberts, L. W., Warner, T. D., Moutier, C., Geppert, C. M. A., & Hammond, K. A. G. (2011). *Are Doctors Who Have Been Ill More Compassionate? Attitudes of Resident Physicians Regarding Personal Health Issues and the Expression of Compassion in Clinical Care.* www.psychosomaticsjournal.org

Schwartz, K. B. (1995, July 16). A patient's story. *The Boston Globe Magazine.* https://www.pointofcarefoundation.org.uk/our-work/schwartz-rounds/

Singer, T., & Klimecki, O. M. (2014). Empathy and compassion. In *Current Biology* (Vol. 24, Issue 18, pp. R875–R878). https://doi.org/10.1016/j.cub.2014.06.054

Smith, J. A. (Interviewer), & Bellitto, C. M. (Guest). (2023, November 21). *How do we make humility important again?* https://greatergood.berkeley.edu/article/item/how_do_we_make_humility_important_again?utm_source=Greater+Good+Science+Center&utm_campaign=c95b22fc4f-EMAIL_CAM-PAIGN_GG_Newsletter_November_21_2023&utm_medium=email&utm_term=0_5ae73e326e-c95b22fc4f-70710255

Spezio, M., Peterson, G., & Roberts, R. C. (2019). Humility as openness to others: Interactive humility in the context of l'Arche. *Journal of Moral Education, 48*(1), 27–46. https://doi.org/10.1080/03057240.2018.1444982

Strauss, C., Lever Taylor, B., Gu, J., Kuyken, W., Baer, R., Jones, F., & Cavanagh, K. (2016). What is compassion and how can we measure it? A review of definitions and measures. *Clinical Psychology Review, 47*, 15–27. https://doi.org/10.1016/j.cpr.2016.05.004

Tutu, D., & Tutu, M. (2014). A world of forgiveness. In D. C. Abrahams (Ed.), *The Book of Forgiving. The Fourfold Path for Healing Ourselves and Our World* (First edition, pp. 213–223). William Collins.

Van Tongeren, D. R., Davis, D. E., Hook, J. N., & Witvliet, C. van O. (2019). Humility. *Current Directions in Psychological Science, 28*(5), 463–468. https://doi.org/10.1177/0963721419850153

What your patient is thinking. (2023). The power of the small stuff. *BMJ,* p2332. https://doi.org/10.1136/bmj.p2332

9 Communication

This chapter talks about the nature of the bio-behavioural signals implicit in communication. These signals are used in an emotional co-regulatory capacity to create safe relationships as the basis for compassion, and form part of the experience of compassion itself.

Behavioural vectors for emotional co-regulation

Patterns of speech, touch, eye gaze and facial expression, as well as the relative position, movement and proximity of one person to another, all function as bio-behavioural signals. Taken together, they comprise an embodied and uniquely sensitive signalling system that is designed to convey compassion or compassionate intent. This signalling system is also capable of communicating a variety of other intentions, depending upon whether or not there is ongoing threat system processing involving SNS reactivity, the amygdala and the pituitary-adrenal axis or oxytocin-opiate-parasympathetic stimulation providing a calming, steadying and encouraging effect.

It is thought that human beings are highly attuned to be able to 'read' and respond to bio-behavioural signals in other people, with no recourse to deliberative thinking because of the relevance of the signals to safety and survival (Porges, 2022). These bio-behavioural signals also have a mutually-influencing effect, and there is a porosity of experience between people. If the threat processing system has been activated and bio-behavioural signals of angry arousal are being emitted by one person, this can trigger the threat processing system and consequent 'fight or flight' or submissive tendencies in another.

The reverse is also possible with the use of intentional bio-behavioural signalling. One person in a state of calm arising from a place of oxytocin-opiate-parasympathetic influence can emotionally co-regulate another person in a state of angry or fearful arousal 'down' to a state of comparative calm by deactivating or suppressing threat processing activity with a calming and steadying presence.

DOI: 10.4324/9781003427247-9

This can and does work as an effective de-escalation technique in some labile situations and is something that some healthcare workers do routinely as part of their role. Emotional co-regulation is known to take place between intimate partners or children and parents (Butler & Randall, 2013), but there is an implicit and sometimes unacknowledged expectation on the part of patients that healthcare personnel will engage with them in an emotional co-regulatory role when they are distressed by health-related states of shame or fear, or both.

Speech

What is said, how it is said and the way that people speak to each other are of importance for the cultivation of compassion and the creation of compassionate health care systems.

It is possible to either activate the threat processing system in another person with harsh words and a judgmental tone or to stimulate oxytocin-opiate-parasympathetic circuitry with a form of words that is supportive and spoken in a gentle tone of voice. Moreover, it is possible to activate either of these two systems in oneself in the same way with a self-focused internal narrative.

Words flagging inclusion and therapeutic interest were found to be associated with positive changes in mood in hospitalised inpatients (Mascaro et al., 2022), and it is possible to denigrate and disempower people with the use of outdated medical language, or alternatively, to uplift and empower them with carefully chosen words (Cox & Fritz, 2022).

Sensitivity to individual words and the subtle nuance that they carry when used in difficult conversations where there are opposing views can help engagement and dialogue (Yeomans et al., 2020) and mitigate the use of speech as a 'power-laden' practice (Dahlke & Hunter, 2020, p. 1). The process of respectful 'turn taking' in conversation itself is an important part of this relational practice. Allowing others to speak rather than 'talking over' other people, either patients or colleagues, requires the conscious and active suppression of speech to allow listening to take place (Porges, 2009). Listening itself signals engagement in the process of co-creating feelings of safety and respect, conditions that are necessary for the expression and experience of compassion within relationships between healthcare personnel and their patients.

There is also a rich transmission of detectable emotions in human vocal expression alone (Simon-Thomas et al., 2009), so it is possible to discern cries of pain from exclamations of excitement and enjoyment without word content. Tone of voice is important in conveying civility, and it is entirely possible to say one thing whilst clearly conveying another (Porath & Pearson, 2015). It is known that the voice broadcasts rich meaning beyond words alone and that meaning is decoded by the brain from the sound of the voice to help understanding and interpretation when there is complexity and ambiguity present in social interactions (Grandjean, 2021).

Focus box 9.1   Choosing speech to convey compassion

(Are the words likely to activate the threat processing system or increase oxytocin-opiate-parasympathetic influence?)

What is the intention behind these words?
Are they kind?
Are they skilful?
Does this need to be said right now?

Touch

The way that people are touched when they are stressed or in pain may either add to their suffering or soothe them by stimulating the oxytocin-opiate-parasympathetic system. Touch of all of the bio-behavioural signals is most strongly associated with the expression of care and compassion, because of the importance of the role of maternal touch in care giving in infancy and early childhood (Goetz et al., 2010). It is known that touch can also convey specific emotions, and massage, for example, provides well-known physiological health benefits in a variety of contexts (Field, 2010). Very brief touch can also convey clear benefits to people who are distressed, and it has been suggested that touch is under-explored in hospital settings when it could help relieve stress at key points in the patient journey (Field, 2010).

The role of many healthcare professionals involves 'procedural touch', that is, touch as part of a clinical task as they carry out the responsibilities associated with their role (Davin et al., 2019, p. e284). Whilst permission is usually sought before procedural touch by healthcare professionals, there is often very little real choice for patients because much of the work of healthcare is necessarily 'body-based'. The pairing of touch with either reassuring speech or frequent reassuring gaze or both, to convey an intentionality of compassion when some pain is caused as part of care, is fundamental to maintaining an ongoing sense of sufficient safety. This form of 'checking in' with the patient also ensures that the threat processing system is not triggered and allows injuries or painful parts of the body to be touched for examination or therapy more easily (Ahlsen & Nilsen, 2022).

Expressive touch has been defined as touch that is unrelated to examination or procedure but is used to signal compassion, concern or interest alone (Davin et al., 2019). Touch, however, both procedural and expressive, is a two-way process or a relational practice in healthcare, and the exercise of power is implicit. Patients are not expected to touch healthcare workers back, and healthcare workers are expected to uphold clear professional boundaries when touch takes place, for example by wearing uniforms and badges that display names and roles in the healthcare organisation concerned (Kelly et al., 2018). Routine touch, for example, handholding by nurses, can be used to convey compassion, but a wide range of other clinicians may also engage in compassionate touch. Compassionate touch has been perceived by some as more complex in the context of caring for people with mental health problems (Kelly et al., 2018) and simpler with other groups of people, for example, the elderly, although misinterpretation, mostly of sexual intent, is often feared (Cocksedge et al., 2013).

Cultural practices and religious beliefs may also influence when and how touch is offered as a compassionate response to suffering (Singh et al., 2018), but the same attunement to the preferences and needs of the individual in the moment is required in addition to any broader knowledge that might serve to guide behaviour.

Gaze and facial expression

The frequency, intensity and duration of eye contact combined with facial expression are equally important in conveying the degree of activation of the threat processing system, or the state of equanimity afforded by oxytocin-opiate-parasympathetic circuitry stimulation. More subtle messaging, however, is also conveyed. A lack of eye contact in healthcare, for example, when staff are completing online notes in a clinic setting, is often interpreted by patients as demonstrating a lack of interest and can contribute to the degradation of the patient-professional partnership. A gentle gaze and a friendly, interested facial expression signal compassionate intent and can generate feelings of connection very briefly or as part of a longer exchange. Patients often mention active listening skills as important in compassion (Patel et al., 2019; Wildbore et al., 2024), and these necessarily include eye contact, facial expression and other body movements, including that of the head.

Body

Body posture, proximity, relative position and movement all matter and certain bio-behavioural signals and combinations of bio-behavioural signals are particularly salient. The intentionality of movement towards others is decoded rapidly, so for example, a sudden lunge made towards another person would likely signal threat. Other rapid, sudden movements like quickly turning or walking away from a potentially aggressive person are known to increase the likelihood of triggering a violent reaction (Porges, 2009), probably either because such a move is interpreted as a sudden termination of the possibility for friendly engagement or strategically it is seen as an opportunity for a successful attack, or a combination of both. Standing over someone to talk to them may be experienced as intimidating, whereas intentionally positioning oneself at the same height as another person is likely to signal less threat and an increased willingness to engage in a friendly way.

Being present and feeling connected

Each of the above behavioural vectors was associated with the experience of compassion by patients in a review of curricula for empathy and compassion training in medicine (Patel et al., 2019). The capacity for the bio-behavioural vectors combined to signal attunement and responsivity, representing 'physician presence and focus', was also discussed in the same study and highlighted as a possible unifying factor for the findings overall (Patel et al., 2019, p. 17). It seems very likely that it is the attuned and responsive nature of the bio-behavioural signalling and associated emotional coregulatory function that takes place as the situation unfolds that is so important and that is experienced as compassion (Halifax, 2012, 2013), rather than the use of any particular behaviours alone.

The capacity to be present and attuned can be enhanced or developed through training, and it is often associated with some degree of mindfulness (see Halifax, 2013 for an example). It is also the case, however, that some members of the workforce will be particularly proficient in using relational skills without any training, the people that Porges (2022) refers to as 'super co-regulators'. The intentional use of the behavioural vectors described in the study by Patel et al. (2019) is an essential component of a process that is co-created between the patient and the healthcare professional. The process affords both physiological benefits mediated by oxytocin-opiate-parasympathetic circuitry and provides a meaningful sense of connection for both the healthcare worker and the patient.

Two skill sets

Offering compassion in healthcare is reliant on two different sets of competencies that are practised alongside each other in different blends according to the needs of the patient as they arise. The first competency is proficiency in using the relational skills for effective emotional co-regulation to convey compassion, and the second competency consists of proficiency in any other profession-specific skills necessary for the care of that particular patient. One of the skills that relates to emotional co-regulation is assessing the extent to which the patient requires or is expecting the healthcare professional to engage with them in order to provide an emotional co-regulatory function. Making an accurate assessment of this need and then meeting that need with skill and sensitivity is essential for the patient to experience the encounter as compassionate. When patients with a range of health conditions were asked in a survey to choose whether or not they preferred competence over compassion in their doctors, patients indicated that the flexible use of both skill sets were desirable in order to effectively help them to navigate changes in their condition and situation as they arose (Heinze et al., 2020).

Focus box 9.2   Emotional co-regulation of states of health-related shame and fear

Is the main function of compassion as described by Porges
Is an expectation of healthcare professionals by patients
Is mediated by the quality of bio-behavioural signalling implicit in
   communication
Is a relational skill

Individual differences

Sometimes, nuanced and unexpected interpretations of any of the bio-behavioural signals or combinations of bio-behavioural signals may be made. This can happen for both members of the healthcare workforce and patients alike. Idiosyncratic interpretations can arise from life experiences that have shaped and tuned receptivity and responsiveness to signals of safety and threat, and this can become problematic at times, depending upon the nature and degree of any distortion present. The use of alcohol and some drugs can alter the interpretation of, or response to, bio-behavioural signals, as can serious illness, both psychological and physical.

Summary points

There is an expectation that healthcare professionals can move smoothly between relational skills and other profession-specific competencies required for patient care

All the behavioural vectors involved in communication can help convey presence and connection

Bodily proximity and position may reinforce unhelpful power relationships between patients and members of the workforce or help to change them

All of the behavioural vectors need to be considered in the context of patient preference

Receptivity to and interpretation of bio-behavioural signals may be influenced by individual differences, illness, alcohol and drugs

References

Ahlsen, B., & Nilsen, A. B. (2022). Getting in touch: Communication in physical therapy practice and the multiple functions of language. *Frontiers in Rehabilitation Sciences, 3*, 1–9.

Butler, E. A., & Randall, A. K. (2013). Emotional coregulation in close relationships. *Emotion Review, 5*(2), 202–210. https://doi.org/10.1177/1754073912451630

Cocksedge, S., George, B., Renwick, S., & Chew-Graham, C. A. (2013). Touch in primary care consultations: Qualitative investigation of doctors' and patients' perceptions. *British Journal of General Practice, 63*(609). https://doi.org/10.3399/bjgp13X665251

Cox, C., & Fritz, Z. (2022). Presenting complaint: Use of language that disempowers patients. *The BMJ*. https://doi.org/10.1136/bmj-2021-066720

Dahlke, S., & Hunter, K. F. (2020). How nurses' use of language creates meaning about healthcare users and nursing practice. *Nursing Inquiry, 27*(3). https://doi.org/10.1111/nin.12346

Davin, L., Thistlethwaite, J., Bartle, E., & Russell, K. (2019). Touch in health professional practice: A review. *Clinical Teacher, 16*(6), 559–564. https://doi.org/10.1111/tct.13089

de Groot, J. H. B., & Smeets, M. A. M. (2017). Human fear chemosignaling: Evidence from a meta-analysis. *Chemical Senses, 42*(8), 663–673. https://doi.org/10.1093/chemse/bjx049

Field, T. (2010). Touch for socioemotional and physical well-being: A review. *Developmental Review, 30*(4), 367–383. https://doi.org/10.1016/j.dr.2011.01.001

Goetz, J. L., Keltner, D., & Simon-Thomas, E. (2010). Compassion: An evolutionary analysis and empirical review. *Psychological Bulletin, 136*(3), 351–374. https://doi.org/10.1037/a0018807

Grandjean, D. (2021). Brain networks of emotional prosody processing. *Emotion Review, 13*(1), 34–43. https://doi.org/10.1177/1754073919898522

Halifax, J. (2012). A heuristic model of enactive compassion. *Current Opinion in Supportive and Palliative Care, 6*(2), 228–235. https://doi.org/10.1097/SPC.0b013e3283530fbe

Halifax, J. (2013). G.R.A.C.E. for nurses: Cultivating compassion in nurse/patient interactions. *Journal of Nursing Education and Practice, 4*(1). https://doi.org/10.5430/jnep.v4n1p121

Heinze, K., Suwanabol, P. A., Vitous, C. A., Abrahamse, P., Gibson, K., Lansing, B., & Mody, L. (2020). A survey of patient perspectives on approach to health care:

Focus on physician competency and compassion. *Journal of Patient Experience*, *7*(6), 1044–1053. https://doi.org/10.1177/2374373520968447

Kelly, M. A., Nixon, L., McClurg, C., Scherpbier, A., King, N., & Dornan, T. (2018). Experience of touch in health care: A meta-ethnography across the health care professions. *Qualitative Health Research*, *28*(2), 200–212. https://doi.org/10.1177/1049732317707726

Mascaro, J. S., Palmer, P. K., Willson, M., Ash, M. J., Florian, M. P., Srivastava, M., Sharma, A., Jarrell, B., Walker, E. R., Kaplan, D. M., Palitsky, R., Cole, S. P., Grant, G. H., & Raison, C. L. (2022). The language of compassion: Hospital chaplains' compassion capacity reduces patient depression via other-oriented, inclusive language. *Mindfulness*. https://doi.org/10.1007/s12671-022-01907-6

Patel, S., Pelletier-Bui, A., Smith, S., Roberts, M. B., Kilgannon, H., Trzeciak, S., & Roberts, B. W. (2019). Curricula for empathy and compassion training in medical education: A systematic review. *PLoS ONE*, *14*(8), 1–25. https://doi.org/10.1371/journal.pone.0221412

Porath, C., & Pearson, C. (2015). The price of incivility. In *HBR's 10 Must Reads. The Price of Incivility: Lack of Respect Hurts Morale - and the Bottom Line* (First edition, pp. 93–104). Harvard Business Review Press.

Porges, S. W. (2009). Reciprocal influences between body and brain in the perception and expression of affect: A polyvagal perspective. In D. Fosha, D. J. Siegel, & M. F. Solomon (Eds.), *The Power of Emotion: Affective Neuroscience, Development, Clinical Practice* (First edition). Norton.

Porges, S. W. (2022). Polyvagal theory: A science of safety. In *Frontiers in Integrative Neuroscience* (Vol. 16). Frontiers Media S.A. https://doi.org/10.3389/fnint.2022.871227

Simon-Thomas, E. R., Keltner, D. J., Sauter, D., Sinicropi-Yao, L., & Abramson, A. (2009). The voice conveys specific emotions: Evidence from vocal burst displays. *Emotion*, *9*(6), 838–846. https://doi.org/10.1037/a0017810

Singh, P., King-Shier, K., & Sinclair, S. (2018). The colours and contours of compassion: A systematic review of the perspectives of compassion among ethnically diverse patients and healthcare providers. In *PLoS ONE* (Vol. 13, Issue 5). Public Library of Science. https://doi.org/10.1371/journal.pone.0197261

Wildbore, E., Bond, C., Timmons, S., Hui, A., & Sinclair, S. (2024). Service users' perspectives on communicating compassion in mental health practice. *Nursing Open*, *11*(11). https://doi.org/10.1002/nop2.70081

Yeomans, M., Minson, J., Collins, H., Chen, F., & Gino, F. (2020). Conversational receptiveness: Improving engagement with opposing views. *Organizational Behavior and Human Decision Processes*, *160*, 131–148. https://doi.org/10.1016/j.obhdp.2020.03.011

10 Practical compassion

This chapter provides a brief recap on the emotional co-regulation role of healthcare professionals and focuses on the application of compassion as an everyday practice. It uses the Cognitive Therapy framework as a means of summarising the salient features that are involved in, and comprise a compassionate response, and suggests a revised definition of compassion for use in health and social care.

The function of compassion is emotional co-regulation for patients

The first role-related competency is for healthcare workers *to bear professional witness to the suffering and vulnerability of the people that they care for, without triggering feelings of health-related shame or fear.* This avoids triggering the threat processing system involving SNS reactivity, the amygdala and the pituitary-adrenal axis (Gilbert, 2014) and uses up metabolic resources that would otherwise be used for healing and restoration (Porges, 2017).

The second role-related competency is for healthcare workers to *intentionally use their professional skills, including those of a relational and communicative nature, to alleviate and prevent suffering, including feelings of health-related shame and fear.* This process actively stimulates the oxytocin-opiate-parasympathetic system to promote feelings of safety and encouragement in the patient and can also lead to feelings of connection and presence between the healthcare professional and the patient. The patient feels that the healthcare worker is available for them; they feel a sense of connection, and this is experienced as compassionate contact. The healthcare worker feels that they are focused and present for the patient, and there is a sense of connection that is pleasing and professionally satisfying. The co-creation of feelings of safety and encouragement and connection and presence constitutes an emotional co-regulation process that is active in both the patient and the healthcare worker simultaneously and is associated with short-term health benefits for both participants in the encounter (Porges, 2017).

DOI: 10.4324/9781003427247-10

> **Focus box 10.1   Emotional co-regulation from the perspective of the healthcare worker**
>
> Firstly, co-creating feelings of safety and encouragement in the patient
>
> Secondly, co-creating mutually experienced feelings of presence and connection, experienced as compassion by patients

Considerations for compassion

Compassion in health and social care, because of the acuity of some situations, will be one of a number of competing priorities that need to be acted upon accordingly. For example, life saving measures and infection control are two important aspects of care that might require consideration before considering compassion. Nonetheless, given the potent effects of compassion in reducing the potential for psychological harm following a life-threatening medical emergency (Moss et al., 2019), exploring the potential to infuse compassion into any aspect of care during acute events when patients might feel especially vulnerable would seem to be particularly worthwhile.

The relational space

Much of the healthcare literature refers to compassion taking place in the 'relational space' between the patient and healthcare provider (e.g., Sinclair et al., 2016). Creating a relational space that is inclusive and fit for compassionate purpose, however, necessarily includes a skilled approach to taking into account any social injustice or identity-based suffering that is present or that emerges within that space as the interaction unfolds. Changes in the perception of interpersonal signs of threat and safety following trauma for example, may need to be navigated sensitively so that the quality of the contact between the healthcare professional and the patient remains one that is conducive to the expression and experience of compassion, respectively.

Connecting with compassion

Notions of common humanity can be helpful in facilitating compassionate action in healthcare workers, but rehearsing exactly how a sense of common humanity will be invoked 'in the moment' is important. This preparation is preferable to waiting for a difficult situation to arise, when action may be more likely to be driven by the prevailing (and likely reactive) mood of the moment (Feldman, 2017) than it is by intention or professional aspirations to uphold compassion as an essential value in healthcare.

Preparing a brief form of words beforehand, for example, 'just like me this person has hopes and fears ...', or a visual image to hold in mind at times of challenge that helps to connect with empathic concern or the intention to be compassionate, can all be helpful. When sufficient safety has been established, sometimes it helps to connect with people who are exhibiting aggressive behaviour by reminding oneself that no one is introduced to violence as a perpetrator. Similarly, it can be recalled that challenging life experiences can shape people, their lives and behaviour in ways that they did not ask for. Other approaches to cultivating compassionate intent are more focused on the healthcare provider, as in re-committing to uphold compassion as an essential value in healthcare or briefly promoting a compassionate self-identity for oneself in the moment, for example, by silently invoking words such as 'may I be of benefit' at appropriate times (see Fernando et al., 2016, p. 340).

Approaching compassion in a conscious and intentional way may be a new way of working for some people, but for other healthcare workers, already proactive in the face of difficult situations or challenging people, it presents an opportunity to affirm and celebrate the skilful nature of their actions. The only requirement is that any cues or prompts used are helpful and do not cause empathic distress in the people that use them. Different prompts and combinations of prompts can be discussed and explored with colleagues to see which resonate most helpfully and the situations that they are most suited to.

Using mindfulness skills in difficult situations

If it is difficult to bring compassion to bear, or the situation is very difficult, it can be helpful to remember that the task in hand is only ever the size of the moment (Feldman, 2012), and since this holds true, it can help things to feel more manageable. On this basis it is possible to approach any situation with a mindful sensitivity to the moment-by-moment nature of its unfolding and to gently adjust the way in which one is relating to the other person or people as necessary. This constitutes in part moving in to a 'growth mindset' (Dweck, 2007) and is helpful in itself, as it involves relating to the difficulty differently, and seeing it as an opportunity to learn rather than a problem to be overcome. This perspective holds the potential to provide a more enjoyable way of engaging with difficult situations since they are the 'growing edge' for developing and practising compassion-related skills. Dweck (2007, p. 255) also suggests

talking directly to a 'fixed mindset' to help with flexibility and movement on difficult issues and makes the very useful point that it is possible
to learn from difficulty until the point at which the difficulty is entirely
blamed on others or it is denied.

In the middle of challenging situations with patients or colleagues,
it is 'perfectly human' to wish that the situation was different, but it is
also futile because the ongoing experience has already emerged to be
exactly what it has become, and there is no turning the clock back. The
headspace invested in the process of struggling with an unwanted reality reduces energetic and attentional resources that might otherwise be
available to explore the potential for a more fruitful approach, including
that of skill development. This is because struggling with an ongoing
unwanted experience tends to activate the threat processing system that
in turn restricts the capacity of the thinking mind to strategies involving avoidance or escape from what is unpleasant. This activation of the
threat processing system simultaneously stifles any oxytocin-opiate-
parasympathetic influence that is associated with flexible thinking, effective problem solving and a physical state conducive to wellbeing.

A mindful noting of any aversive responses, however, including the
presence of thoughts, emotions, physical sensations and impulses to act,
is useful to provide perspective. The process of creating space and stepping back using a STOP practice (e.g., Ciarrochi et al., 2014, p. 10) then
further allows for the possibility of something more considered and compassionate to be enacted once the connection to values, motivation or
intention has been re-established (see Focus box 10.2 and Figure 10.1).
To let go of the struggle (Feldman, 2012) is in itself an act of agency and
self-compassion and an important step in deactivating the threat processing system. This self-compassion also helps to bring the oxytocin-
opiate-parasympathetic system online more fully to further restore a
sense of balance and confidence in one's own capacity to handle the
situation with skill and professional integrity.

Focus box 10.2   The STOP practice

S. Steady and ground yourself. Feel into the solidity of the body.
T. Take note. Notice physical sensations, thoughts, emotions and
   action impulses.
O. Open up to them. Allow them to be there, but step back from
   them.
P. Pursue a compassionate choice

```
┌─────────────────────────┐                              ┌─────────────────────────┐
│ Acting ineffectively and│                              │   Acting skilfully and  │
│    uncompassionately    │                              │    compassionately      │
└─────────────────────────┘                              └─────────────────────────┘
```

┌─────────────────────────┐   ┌─────────────────────┐   ┌─────────────────────────┐
│   Impeding factors   │   │   Make a choice   │   │   Supporting factors   │
│   Automaticity &   │   │   STOP practice   │   │   Recalling intention │
│   reactivity   │   │ Draw on the supporting│ │ Identification with all of│
└─────────────────────────┘   │   factors   │   │   humanity   │
                               └─────────────────────┘   │   Feeling into a   │
                                                          │   compassionate   │
                                                          │ professional/personal   │
                                                          │   identity   │
                                                          └─────────────────────────┘

                          ┌──────────────────────────────┐
                          │ Challenging situation with patient│
                          │   or colleague   │
                          └──────────────────────────────┘

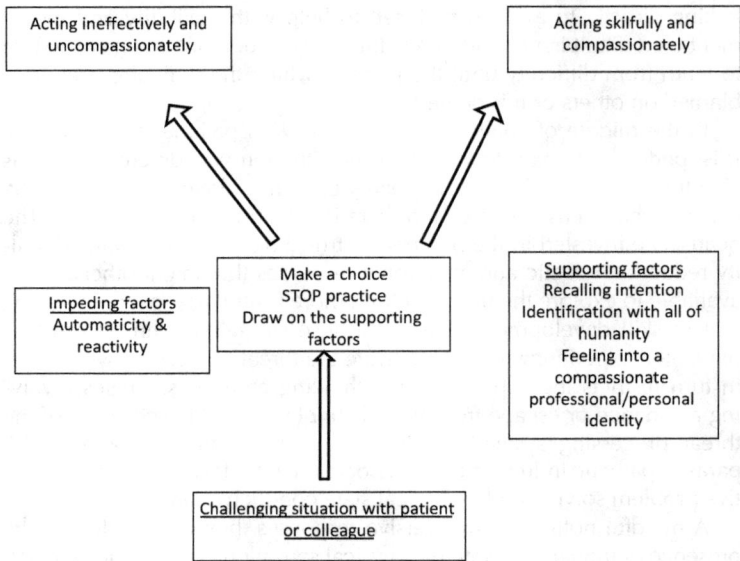

Figure 10.1 The compassionate choice point.

Figure 10.1 is adapted from The Weight Escape: How to Stop Dieting and Start Living by Joseph Ciarrochi, Ann Bailey and Russ Harris. Copyright ©2014 by Ann Bailey, Joseph Ciarrochi and Russ Harris. Reprinted by arrangement with The Permissions Company, LLC on behalf of Shambhala Publications, Inc., Boulder, Colorado, shambhala.com.

It is not being suggested that any of these skills are acquired in the service of tolerating the intolerable. Instead, mindfulness is learnt to strengthen confidence in managing difficult situations with compassion, along with developing the capacity to understand and discern the conditions that are needed to do that. Importantly, practising compassion in a healthy way is always inclusive of the needs of oneself (Feldman, 2017), including that of being sufficiently safe, as well as any needs that the patient also might present.

Presence and connection

Patients and the people that are close to them seek authenticity, presence and connection from the healthcare professionals that they have contact with, and this is particularly the case if there is very serious illness or high levels of distress or vulnerability. Presence and connection appear to be properties of relationship that have a strong and beneficial emotional co-regulatory effect and are most often experienced as compassion by patients. Much compassion in physical health settings is expressed through specific procedures that are learnt through training and that either alleviate or prevent suffering, for example, a surgical procedure to restore function or physiotherapy exercises to the same end. Describing and teaching the process of emotional co-regulation with another person, however, is more subtle.

All of the available evidence suggests, however, that states of safety and encouragement that then form the basis for presence and connection as the experience of compassion are co-created between people. The bio-behavioural signalling behaviours involved in facial expression, eye gaze, speech, voice tone, body movement and proximity on the part of the healthcare worker (Patel et al., 2019) are used to regulate the emotional state of the patient. A mindful attunement to one's own internal state is thought to increase sensitivity to the internal state of others (Halifax, 2013; Price & Hooven, 2018), and this in turn increases the capacity to respond sensitively to another. An undistracted focus on the patient lends itself to a sense of presence and connection from both a patient and healthcare worker perspective (Patel et al., 2019; Sinclair et al., 2016). So, for example, the healthcare worker is not able to be present with a patient if they are distracted by thoughts of blood results to be chased or very sick patients to be seen and cared for.

Being present, is not a performative, self-conscious or effortful way of relating to the patient on the part of the healthcare professional. There is a sense of authenticity that emerges from an absence of the need to become involved in a simultaneous process of curating the professional self that detracts from the quality of the contact in the encounter. There is also a sharing of the experience that 'breaks any sense of existential isolation' for both the healthcare professional and the patient (Greenberg, 2007, p. 54), and whilst it makes for meaningful contact in the encounter, it is neither 'heavy' nor intimidating for either participant in the interaction. Overall, there is far less reliance on any profession-specific knowledge but an increased willingness to trust in the healing power of human presence and connection as 'enough' and what is required in that moment.

Importantly, cultivating connection with patients does not mean over-involvement or over-disclosure, although to some extent such boundaries often relate to a combination of personal confidence and professional experience. Instead, for each individual there is a process of exploring an appropriate and authentic expression of compassion that is in alignment with professional boundaries and that consists of a blend of relational skills for emotional co-regulation along with any

Table 10.1 The experience of presence and connection compared with emotional contagion for the healthcare worker

Presence and connection	Emotional contagion
Pleasant, satisfying emotional experience	Unpleasant, unwanted emotional experience
Sense of effective professional self is retained	Erosion of sense of effective professional self
Sense of physical self, grounded and steady	Lack of contact with body/overwhelmed by physical sensations
Behavioural engagement	Behavioural withdrawal (or wish to escape)
Personal boundaries intact	Patient distress is felt as an intrusion beyond personal boundaries

other professional competencies required for the care of the patient at that time (Table 10.1).

Expressive and procedural compassion

Whilst the terms expressive and procedural have been used in connection with the bio-behavioural signal of interpersonal touch (Davin et al., 2019), these terms can also usefully be applied to compassion itself. Expressive compassion involves addressing suffering through bio-behavioural means, for example, talking to someone about their distress or expressing compassion through facial expression and gaze, alone. Procedural compassion is reliant on conveying compassion to relieve suffering through the quality of task-related contact, and that in practice often involves touch, for example, bathing or feeding someone very attentively or inserting a cannula as gently as possible. Both expressive and procedural compassion often take place within the same healthcare encounter, for example, engaging someone in conversation first, before going on to change a dressing.

Opportunities for compassion

Being 'in relationship' with another person is a uniquely human experience. Engaging with another person offers an opportunity for the co-creation of a mutually benefical, caring and compassionate relationship through means of embodied and evolved bio-behavioural signalling systems. Importantly, these bio-behavioural systems evolved especially for being 'in relationship' with strangers in novel situations in order to assess threat and to explore and facilitate the possibility of friendly engagement.

On this basis it is clear that it is not necessary for a patient and healthcare worker to know each other well in order for the healthcare worker to co-create and establish a relationship of safety and encouragement with the patient, quickly and effectively.

Healthcare encounters may take place in a physical location with both participants present, for example, a room in a care home, or in a virtual space serviced with 'live' video capability, or speaking on a cell phone. Each of these modalities are employed by healthcare workers to connect with patients and each offers either access to the words and quality of voice used by the healthcare worker and, in some cases, facial expression. Both healthcare professionals and patients often prefer to be in the same room as each other, but it is possible to co-create relationships of safety and encouragement as well as establish presence and connection in virtual spaces, too.

What compassion isn't

Undertaking tasks that lie outside the remit of their role but benefit patients may be a sign of institutional problems that frontline staff feel compelled to compensate for (Gillespie & Reader, 2021; Papadopoulos et al., 2017). Whilst these actions are sometimes spoken about by patients as indicating a compassionate attitude and appreciated as such, they can represent something else much less desirable. Unfortunately they are usually a further pressure on already 'stretched' members of the healthcare workforce who see the shortcomings in the care they are trying to provide.

The Cognitive Therapy model as a summary for compassionate practice

Compassion is an action-based, interpersonal and iterative process that unfolds on a moment-by-moment basis, but the dimensions of experience involved for the healthcare worker can usefully be summarised and represented by a Cognitive Therapy framework (see Figure 10.1).

In the *physiological dimension*, the embodied experience of oxytocin-opiate-parasympathetic stimulation as part of expressing compassion or readiness to express compassion is one of feeling grounded and steady, available for, and connected to the patient.

Within the *thought dimension*, there are a number of questions that are active and 'alive' as part of an ongoing inquiry throughout the encounter and that help to inform the appropriate and attuned expression of compassionate action. The questions in the cognitive dimension can be distilled into one: What is required in this moment?

Focus box 10.3   Questions to help inform the expression of compassionate action

What is required in this moment ?

Does the intention to be compassionate need to be renewed?
What function of compassion is being fulfilled here (fear/shame)?
What quality of compassion is appropriate here (gentle/assertive)?
What direction of compassion is needed here (other/self)?
What does compassion sound like/look like right now (behaviour)?
Are there other pressing clinical concerns that need to be accommodated right now?
How is inclusivity being taken care of right now?

Patient-focused feelings of care and concern arise in the *emotional dimension* and can include empathic concern that is intentionally generated. Other emotions that might arise include feelings of personal or professional satisfaction and confidence in one's own skills.

The *behavioural dimension* includes the use of a dual skill set that can be blended as required, in response to the needs of the patient. Firstly, relational skills for the effective emotional co-regulation of health-related shame and fear and the co-creation of feelings of safety and encouragement, and secondly, competency in any other profession-specific skills required for the care of the patient.

Shifts in any one dimension of experience for the healthcare worker can influence the other domains for better or worse and can also impact the patient experience. So, for example, if there is a lack of knowledge about a profession-specific competency required to deal effectively with a situation (the behavioural dimension), this becomes stressful for the healthcare worker. As a result, there may be a loss of presence and connection with the patient as the threat processing system is activated in the healthcare worker. This is because the focus has moved away from the relationship with the patient and any procedural compassion to something essential but more peripheral than the co-creation of a compassionate relationship (Figure 10.2).

A revised definition of compassion in health and social care

Strauss and colleagues (2016, p. 26) offer a general definition of compassion including five elements: 'recognising suffering in others; understanding the common humanity of this suffering; feeling emotionally

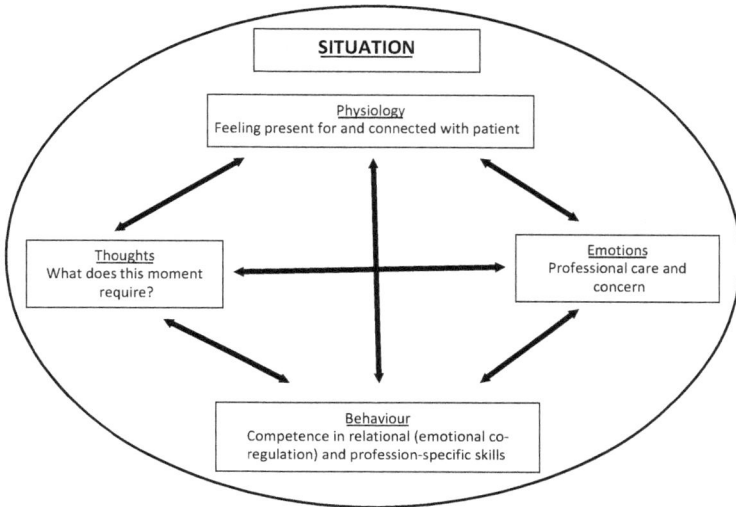

Figure 10.2 The Cognitive Therapy model as a summary of the dimensions of compassionate practice. Adapted with permission of Christine A Padesky, PhD. © 1986 Center for Cognitive Therapy, Newport Beach, CA.

connected with the person who is suffering; tolerating difficult feelings that may arise [and] acting or being motivated to act to help the person'. Their definition has been elaborated and expanded upon to apply more explicitly to the context of health and social care given the function of compassion as explored in this text (see Focus box 10.4).

The prevention of suffering (Gilbert, 2019) is an important component of compassion in healthcare and has been added where relevant. Whilst it is the case that some healthcare personnel are motivated by identifying with all of humanity to support a compassionate practice, others may find different ways of connecting with the intention to be compassionate, for example, calling to mind a sense of professional integrity or self-identity that also demands an inclusive compassion. Both motivation and intention arising from empathic concern are accommodated in the suggested definition below. Emphasis is also placed on the recognition and active management of distress on the part of the healthcare provider on exposure to suffering. The relational and behavioural nature of compassion ('contingent and emergent') is made explicit in definitions developed by Halifax (2012, p. 228); Lown & MacIntosh (2014); Sinclair et al. (2016) and so has been included, along with reference to the two distinct skill sets required for compassion in the context of healthcare.

Focus box 10.4   A revised definition of compassion in health and social care

The anticipation **or** recognition of suffering

Awareness **and** active management of any distress associated with exposure to suffering on the part of the healthcare worker

The motivation **or** intention to prevent **or** alleviate anticipated or ongoing suffering

Engaging in responsive, compassionate action using **either** relational skills (for emotional co-regulation) **or** other professional-specific competencies **or** an appropriate blend of both to prevent **or** alleviate suffering

---

Summary points

A state of safety and encouragement is the basis for feelings of presence and connection to arise

Preparing in advance how to approach difficult situations when compassion is called for is helpful

Finding opportunities to provide emotional co-regulation for patients in acute situations is worthwhile

Opportunities for compassionate emotional co-regulation exist wherever there are possibilities for the exchange of bio-behavioural signalling

A definition of compassion in health and social care needs to be health and social care specific and include a dual skill set

References

Ciarrochi, J., Bailey, A., & Harris, R. (2014). *The Weight Escape: How to Stop Dieting and Start Living* (First edition). Shambhala Publications.

Davin, L., Thistlethwaite, J., Bartle, E., & Russell, K. (2019). Touch in health professional practice: A review. *Clinical Teacher*, 16(6), 559–564. https://doi.org/10.1111/tct.13089

Dev, V., Fernando, A. T., Kirby, J. N., & Consedine, N. S. (2019). Variation in the barriers to compassion across healthcare training and disciplines: A cross-sectional study of doctors, nurses, and medical students. *International Journal of Nursing Studies*, 90, 1–10. https://doi.org/10.1016/j.ijnurstu.2018.09.015

Dweck, C. S. (2007). *Mindset. The New Psychology of Success* (Updated edition). Ballantine.

Feldman, C. (2012). *Opening Talk for Origins and Applications of Mindfulness: MBCT/MBSR Retreat*. Dharma Seed.

Feldman, C. (2015). Where does it all go wrong? In *Dharma Seed*. Dharma Seed.

Feldman, C. (2017). Compassion. In *Boundless Heart. The Buddha's Path of Kindness, Compassion, Joy and Equanimity* (First edition). Shambhala.

Fernando, A. T., Arroll, B., & Consedine, N. S. (2016). Enhancing compassion in general practice: It's not all about the doctor. In *British Journal of General Practice* (Vol. 66, Issue 648, pp. 340–341). Royal College of General Practitioners. https://doi.org/10.3399/bjgp16X685741

Gilbert, P. (2014). The origins and nature of compassion focused therapy. *British Journal of Clinical Psychology, 53*(1), 6–41. https://doi.org/10.1111/bjc.12043

Gilbert, P. (2019). Explorations into the nature and function of compassion. *Current Opinion in Psychology, 28*, 108–114. https://doi.org/https://doi.org/10.1016/j.copsyc.2018.12.002

Gillespie, A., & Reader, T. W. (2021). Identifying and encouraging high-quality healthcare: An analysis of the content and aims of patient letters of compliment. *BMJ Quality & Safety, 30*(6), 484–492. https://doi.org/10.1136/bmjqs-2019-010077

Greenberg, L. (2007). Emotion in the therapeutic relationship in emotion-focused therapy. In P. Gilbert & R. Leahy (Eds.), *The Therapeutic Relationship in the Cognitive Behavioral Psychotherapies* (First edition, pp. 43–62). Routledge.

Halifax, J. (2012). A heuristic model of enactive compassion. In *Current Opinion in Supportive and Palliative Care* (Vol. 6, Issue 2, pp. 228–235). https://doi.org/10.1097/SPC.0b013e3283530fbe

Halifax, J. (2013). G.R.A.C.E. for nurses: Cultivating compassion in nurse/patient interactions. *Journal of Nursing Education and Practice, 4*(1). https://doi.org/10.5430/jnep.v4n1p121

Lown, B., & MacIntosh, S. (2014). *Recommendations from a Conference on Advancing Compassionate, Person-and Family-Centered Care Through Interprofessional Education for Collaborative Practice*. https://www.theschwartzcenter.org/media/FINAL-Triple-C-Conference-Recommendations-Report.pdf

Moss, J., Roberts, M. B., Shea, L., Jones, C. W., Kilgannon, H., Edmondson, D. E., Trzeciak, S., & Roberts, B. W. (2019). Healthcare provider compassion is associated with lower PTSD symptoms among patients with life-threatening medical emergencies: A prospective cohort study. *Intensive Care Medicine, 45*(6), 815–822. https://doi.org/10.1007/s00134-019-05601-5

Papadopoulos, I., Taylor, G., Ali, S., Aagard, M., Akman, O., Alpers, L. M., Apostolara, P., Biglete-Pangilinan, S., Biles, J., García, Á. M., González-Gil, T., Koulouglioti, C., Kouta, C., Krepinska, R., Kumar, B. N., Lesińska-Sawicka, M., Diaz, A. L. L., Malliarou, M., Nagórska, M., ... Zorba, A. (2017). Exploring nurses' meaning and experiences of compassion: An international online survey involving 15 countries. *Journal of Transcultural Nursing, 28*(3), 286–295. https://doi.org/10.1177/1043659615624740

Patel, S., Pelletier-Bui, A., Smith, S., Roberts, M. B., Kilgannon, H., Trzeciak, S., & Roberts, B. W. (2019). Curricula for empathy and compassion training in medical education: A systematic review. *PLoS ONE, 14*(8), 1–25. https://doi.org/10.1371/journal.pone.0221412

Porges, S. W. (2017). Vagal pathways: Portals to compassion. In E. M. Seppala, E. Simon-Thomas, S. L. Brown, M. C. Worline, C. D. Cameron, & J. R. Doty (Eds.), *The Oxford Handbook of Compassion Science* (pp. 189–202). Oxford University Press.

Price, C. J., & Hooven, C. (2018). Interoceptive awareness skills for emotion regulation: Theory and approach of mindful awareness in body-oriented therapy (MABT). *Frontiers in Psychology, 9*(MAY). https://doi.org/10.3389/fpsyg.2018.00798

Sinclair, S., McClement, S., Raffin-Bouchal, S., Hack, T. F., Hagen, N. A., McConnell, S., & Chochinov, H. M. (2016). Compassion in health care: An empirical model. *Journal of Pain and Symptom Management, 51*(2), 193–203. https://doi.org/10.1016/j.jpainsymman.2015.10.009

Strauss, C., Lever Taylor, B., Gu, J., Kuyken, W., Baer, R., Jones, F., & Cavanagh, K. (2016). What is compassion and how can we measure it? A review of definitions and measures. *Clinical Psychology Review, 47*, 15–27. https://doi.org/10.1016/j.cpr.2016.05.004

11 Growing compassion in healthcare organisations

Compassion belongs everywhere in health and social care. There is nowhere in any healthcare system that it is inappropriate to raise the profile of compassion to improve its practice, given the importance it has for patient safety and healing, and staff well-being. This chapter explores the possibilities for growing interest in the science and practice of compassion in healthcare organisations.

Working with existing systems and structures

Flagging compassion as an essential value within the frameworks of existing meetings and processes can be a practical way forward. This may be as simple as asking for compassion to be included as an agenda item so that it receives consideration as part of a new initiative and is not forgotten; a brief presentation about the saliency of compassion in healthcare to keep compassion 'alive'; or as part of an evaluative process. There are validated measures of compassion that are available for use in healthcare, and the items on the questionnaires can be used to inform and focus discussions about important aspects of improving services for patients, even if the measures themselves are not used in any other way.

There will always be a 'compassion perspective' in any patient-related discussion, process or meeting, and the skill is in locating where it lies and how best to address it; if the meeting relates to staff, there will also be implications for the way that relationships between members of the workforce are supported to provide compassionate care to patients. Some staff members may have specialist knowledge or skills or wish to use compassion as a focus for an audit of some sort, but it is important that they do not become isolated or begin to feel that they bear the burden for improving compassionate care in their area. Interested individuals from different work areas could be encouraged to 'buddy up' for support and to generate and support ongoing interest in compassion across their organisation.

DOI: 10.4324/9781003427247-11

Including an appropriate level of information on the function of compassion for all members of the workforce who have contact with patients on a routine basis as part of their role is important and likely to be well received (Howick et al., 2024). Reception staff in particular are usually the first point of contact with people who may be anxious or who are irritable about having to wait to be seen and therefore have a particular role in emotional co-regulation. Understanding more about the function of compassion and the way that relatively brief interactions can intentionally and effectively co-create relationships of safety and friendliness transcends the idea of a 'customer care' approach in a way that can pique interest and help to improve skills and confidence in an interesting and satisfying way. For volunteers who assist with wayfinding in hospitals or those who provide meal time or outpatient support, for example, might also find additional information on compassion interesting and enjoyable to learn as well as increasing their own sense of involvement in their volunteering work.

Taking care of working relationships

Sensitivity to the quality of working relationships in the face of current challenges is essential. Being surrounded by colleagues who send out bio-behavioural signals indicating collegiality, warmth and support can offer a very large measure of protection for well-being in staff members in stressful situations. Friendly and approachable senior leadership and management figures are a welcome presence, and their skills in emotional co-regulation can help to offset any sense of threat and anxiety provoked by intense work pressures, including fears of unjustified blame and censure if crises arise.

It is also the case that many areas or teams will have healthcare workers among their number who are already 'super co-regulator[s]' (Porges, 2022, p. 11) and proficient in the relational aspects of care and co-working. Such people are often known and respected for these qualities and stand out as the colleagues who seem to be able to 'read' people well, help to diffuse tensions with their exceptional emotional co-regulation capacity and who are kind and helpful in difficult situations of all varieties.

Using mindfulness skills to develop an appreciation of the moment-by-moment nature of interactions with work colleagues can help to defuse damaging disagreements sometimes seen between co-workers, teams, and professions in healthcare before they become entrenched. Understanding some of these disagreements as driven by competitive social mentalities that are common and easily triggered given overly pressurised circumstances may also have a positive contribution to make in addressing them. Within these situations, blame can recede in favour of restoring relationships and changing modifiable factors to facilitate resolution. Interpersonal conflicts between staff are usually in themselves a cause of suffering for those immediately involved, and the negative effects can ripple out to impact others around them, including patients.

Compassion focused meetings

Schwartz Rounds take place in healthcare facilities around the globe (currently in the UK, Republic of Ireland, Canada, US, Australia and New Zealand), and the rounds are a powerful means of supporting staff to provide compassionate care to patients. The Rounds focus on the emotional impact of caring for patients, and they are based on the premise that feelings of stress and isolation experienced by staff are reduced by talking about them with other staff members.

The format of the rounds themselves and the roles that people take within the rounds are fixed to ensure replicability and for quality assurance purposes. Each organisation has a steering group and the composition of the steering group is made up of a variety of professions and representatives from different and key departments across the healthcare organisation concerned.

Compassion circles (Clark et al., 2022) are reported to be less structured and less resource intensive than Schwartz Rounds and can be set up more spontaneously as a result. The Circles have a greater focus on self-compassion, and verbal participation by all attendees is expected. This is in contrast with Schwartz Rounds, where speaking by audience members is encouraged but there is no expectation that any staff members other than the story tellers and facilitators need to speak. Because the Circles are less formulaic than Schwartz Rounds, however, there may be a greater skill level required on the part of the facilitator on the day, depending upon the nature of the discussion that unfolds.

Balint groups run by the Balint Society operate in the UK, Europe and North America. They are usually run for and facilitated by workers in primary care. Balint groups provide another supportive setting in which any healthcare professional can attend and discuss their emotions in relation to patients, including those of difficulties with compassion or any matter arising from compassion related contact.

Those members of the workforce who are involved in running or attending Schwartz Rounds, Compassion Circles and Balint groups would appear to be natural allies in raising the profile of compassion across organisations. Wherever there is flexibility and the possibility of people meeting together, brief reflective or mindfulness exercises could be used in order for all staff to 'refresh' or 'get in touch' with compassionate intentions. It may be appropriate to introduce such processes at the beginning of steering groups for Schwartz Rounds or other administrative meetings for the Balint groups or Compassion Circles in order to ensure that relationships between supporting individuals and infrastructure are held with as much care and attention as the Rounds, Circles and groups themselves.

Any increase in compassion-related focus and activity in organisations could serve to encourage the development of multi-professional compassion special interest groups, in addition to any Rounds, Circles and groups. Interested individuals from different work areas could be encouraged to 'buddy up' for support and to generate and support ongoing interest in compassion across their organisation.

Invited speakers, online resources and journal papers on the science and practice of compassion could all become a clear focus for meetings with dates planned and publicised well in advance. Virtual gatherings ensure the efficient use of time and facilitate people from one part of the organisation in meeting those from another, including senior leadership figures, to ensure that any efforts are appropriately encouraged and sustained. Group members could also informally support the work of Schwartz Rounds, for example, helping to find story tellers in their local work area and putting them in touch with members of the Schwartz team.

Reverse mentoring schemes

The reverse mentoring scheme as adopted by some UK healthcare organisations (e.g., Raza & Onyesoh, 2020) has as an explicit aim the disruption and reversal of systems and structures that maintain racial inequity, and compassion is already included as an integral component of the framework (see Johnson, 2018). In a study examining the qualities of nominated exemplar allies for underrepresented and marginalised groups in the workplace, compassion, intellectual humility, self-awareness and desire for human interconnectedness all emerged as strong values motivating those who had chosen to become allies (Warren & Warren, 2021). Given the central positioning of compassion and related values within these initiatives, enhancing and emphasising the compassion components of reverse mentoring and allyship programmes with brief compassion meditations could offer further benefits for physical well-being (Schültke et al., 2023) and social connectedness (Kok & Singer, 2017). Organisations could begin to explore the possibility with people about to join the scheme and obtain the views on feasibility from past mentees and mentors.

Recruitment and appraisal

Interviews for prospective staff might also include questions designed to test knowledge about compassion (McClelland & Vogus, 2021) that are appropriate to role and seniority. Sample questions might include:

What is the function of compassion in healthcare? What do patients want when they say that they want compassionate care? How does communication work in compassion? Tell me about the two neurophysiological systems that are thought to be involved in compassion.

Including compassion-related objectives or education as part of an 'onboarding' process and then at regular intervals in appraisal systems for staff may also help to maintain compassion as a high-profile value in the health and social care sector. Professional guidelines for many workers espouse compassion as an important value (e.g., Chartered Society of Physiotherapy, 2019; Nursing and Midwifery Council, 2018), but other priorities and pressures may erode the impetus to keep learning about the science and practice of compassion as it develops, if it is not given continued prominence.

Supervision, teaching and mentoring

Brief compassion-related exercises, reflections and meditations to contact compassionate intentions are enjoyable and valuable ways of upholding compassion as an essential value in healthcare and can easily be integrated within all patient-focused educational opportunities. Techniques that involve rehearsing compassionate responses to patients in the imagination may be well worth exploring in healthcare (Wilson-Mendenhall et al., 2022) and could be incorporated into training and supervision, both in individual and group formats. These exercises include generating sensitivity to the sensory quality of the interaction, connecting to positive feelings of care and concern and imagining the specificity of the compassionate action. Connecting with and re-experiencing a 'compassionate moment' with a patient or colleague in supervision helps to stimulate the oxytocin-opiate-parasympathetic system and the growing embodiment of oneself as a compassionate professional.

It has also been suggested that training staff using virtual reality may be a powerful tool in increasing empathy towards severely behaviourally disturbed people suffering with psychiatric disorders and thus reducing rates of seclusion and restraint (Riches et al., 2022).

Clearly, increased attention to the relational skills involved in the emotional co-regulation of fear and shame is essential in any communication training initiatives for members of the healthcare workforce.

New directions in improving compassionate care

Humility in work relationships, both at the leadership level (Kelemen et al., 2023) and the individual level (Lehmann et al., 2022), promotes psychological safety and is known to mediate staff engagement, well-being and creativity. Within healthcare settings, humility is known to be associated with positive patient experiences, improved health outcomes and effective teamwork (see Michalec, 2023; Michalec et al., 2024; West, 2021). Recently it has been proposed that teaching an 'inclusive compassion' and common humanity (Osei-Tutu, 2024) could improve compassionate care and that teaching humility itself (Michalec, 2023; Reynolds et al., 2023) could also confer considerable benefits for patients.

It has been argued that strongly hierarchical organisations should reflect on the possible benefits of becoming more collaborative as a way of allowing compassionate working to flourish (Pavlova et al., 2022), and compassion itself has been described as a 'potential equaliser of power' (Pavlova et al., 2024, p. 10). Interprofessional education is thought to reduce unhelpful professional 'tribalism' (Kauff et al., 2023, p. 04), and sharing experiences of compassion specifically between different professionals may be useful for all concerned (Dev et al., 2019). Whilst Schwartz Rounds already function to share the experience and challenges of compassion between different health and social care professionals (Maben et al., 2021), this is an idea that could usefully be developed in specificity and formalised further. For example, a locally-based multi-professional compassion special interest group, as mentioned previously, would provide another forum for exploring compassion as a professional practice and to share the skill sets and ideas that people use to cope when it becomes difficult to respond compassionately and what the enabling factors are thought to be when things go well, despite evident challenges.

Radical change in most healthcare systems is thought to be essential, however, if the status and practice of compassion in health and social care are to be transformed (e.g., Howick et al., 2024; Lown, 2021). The pressures that all healthcare systems are under and the consequent adverse effects on the people that work in them are well known; distress is commonly caused by workplace pressure that is often uncontrollable, unpredictable and experienced very acutely. Unfortunately, over stretched and vulnerable staff who may be in need of compassion themselves are less able to attend to the needs of their distressed and vulnerable patients.

Compassion training

There are currently several compassion training courses that are designed to support staff to deliver compassionate care to patients (Jazaieri et al., 2013; Knox & Franco, 2022; Neff et al., 2020; Sinclair et al., 2024). The courses are developed by expert researchers and clinicians in the field; all of the courses are multi-component in nature and are intended to be taught by specialist teachers. Each course has a good evidence base and consists of a series of experiential exercises or meditation practices designed to cultivate different qualities and perspectives known to be associated with compassion. Mindfulness skills, cultivating a compassionate self, widening the circle of care and concern for compassion and developing self-compassion are all common themes within the courses.

The ability to offer oneself compassion is thought to be one of a number of important skills that facilitate offering compassion to others, and as with mindfulness, can be used 'in the moment' to support oneself. Professor Kristin Neff has a number of free resources on self-compassion on her website, Self-Compassion.org, including free introductory sessions to self-compassion. The Compassion Institute is another US-based, non-profit organisation that offers free resources and has information about compassion in the context of health and social care. Professor Paul Gilbert's Compassionate Mind Foundation website also has some free resources available.

Formal compassion training has been shown to result in increases in empathy and feelings of connection with common humanity greater than those in mindfulness trainings alone (Brito-Pons et al., 2018; Jazaieri et al., 2014). It has also been suggested that the enhanced availability or accessibility of empathy and compassion that staff report following compassion training may also help working relationships between healthcare professionals when conflict arises (Klimecki, 2019). People who see their colleagues, trained or not, being compassionate to patients are provided with a direct opportunity to observe behaviour that they can then adopt and adapt, but also benefit from an uplift in mood as a result, and this effect alone is thought to predispose them to act compassionately in turn (Rodrigues Saturn, 2017).

For healthcare staff who are either not able to access compassion training courses, or who do not wish to, it is still possible to explore some of the information about compassion as well as some of the meditation practices included in the courses and to read about the science behind them. The Greater Good Science Centre website, affiliated with the University of Calfornia at Berkeley, has a searchable catalogue of free meditations that can be accessed and used by anyone.

Some kinds of brief compassion-related meditations (those concerned with sending good wishes to others, rather than focused on suffering per se) appear to reduce bias towards others considered as 'out-group' members in experimental studies (Kang et al., 2014), including those considered as outsiders on the basis of race (Stell & Farsides, 2016). More generally this class of meditation has also been found to increase a sense of connection with other people (Hutcherson et al., 2008). Well-wishing meditations have been found to generate positive emotions in the people who practice them (Fredrickson et al., 2008; Zeng et al., 2015), and so these may be of value to healthcare providers as part of a strategy to maintain well-being.

The use of compassion-focused imagery alone may be effective in cultivating self-compassion, although the emergence of self-critical thinking in response to a stand-alone and otherwise unsupported intervention may be problematic for some participants (Maner & Morris, 2019).

Whilst practising compassion has benefits in itself, it is helpful to know other ways of resourcing oneself beyond regular exercise and getting enough sleep that also nourish the capacity to offer compassion. Gratitude practices are thought to have a number of personal and prosocial benefits (Allen, 2018), and there is a mutually reinforcing effect of humility and gratitude (Kruse et al., 2014). Expressing gratitude, even for very small things, as a sense of appreciation arises can be a spontaneous way to make momentary connections with others that are uplifting and support well-being (Frederickson, 2013). There is also a strong relationship between awe and humility and feeling more connected to other people (Stellar et al., 2018), and time spent outside in nature can contribute to feelings of awe, although it also has other benefits of its own (Nutsford et al., 2016; White et al., 2019). Further information and some reflective practices to cultivate awe, gratitude and well-being at work can be found by visiting the Greater Good Science Centre website.

Summary points

Compassion 'belongs' everywhere in health and social care organisations
    Brief 'touch in' points for reminders of and reflections on compassion should be included in teaching and supervision for healthcare workers
    Compassion touch in points should be introduced at multi-professional and senior level meetings
    Health and social care organisations can try to increase and diversify compassion-related interest and activity alongside Schwartz Rounds or other compassion-related groups if they run them
    There are courses designed for healthcare workers to deepen the understanding and practice of compassion

References

Allen, S. (2018). *The Science of Gratitude*. Greater Good Science Center.

Brito-Pons, G., Campos, D., & Cebolla, A. (2018). Implicit or explicit compassion? Effects of compassion cultivation training and comparison with mindfulness-based stress reduction. *Mindfulness, 9*, 1494–1508.

Chartered Society of Physiotherapy. (2019). *Code of Members' Professional Values and Behaviour*. Chartered Society of Physiotherapy.

Clark, M., Bradley, A., Simms, L., Waites, B., Scott, A., Jones, C., Dodd, P., Howell, T., & Tinsley, G. (2022). Cultivating compassion through compassion circles: Learning from experience in mental health care in the NHS. *The Journal of Mental Health Training, Education, and Practice*, *17*(1), 73–86. https://doi.org/https://doi.org/10.1108/JMHTEP-03-2021-0030

Dev, V., Fernando, A. T., Kirby, J. N., & Consedine, N. S. (2019). Variation in the barriers to compassion across healthcare training and disciplines: A cross-sectional study of doctors, nurses, and medical students. *International Journal of Nursing Studies*, *90*, 1–10. https://doi.org/10.1016/j.ijnurstu.2018.09.015

Frederickson, B. L. (2013). What love is. In *Love 2.0. Creating Health and Happiness in Moments of Connection* (pp. 15–38). Plume.

Fredrickson, B. L., Cohn, M. A., Coffey, K. A., Pek, J., & Finkel, S. M. (2008). Open hearts build lives: Positive emotions, induced through loving-kindness meditation, build consequential personal resources. *Journal of Personality and Social Psychology*, *95*(5), 1045–1062. https://doi.org/10.1037/a0013262

Howick, J., de Zulueta, P., & Gray, M. (2024). Beyond empathy training for practitioners: Cultivating empathic healthcare systems and leadership. In *Journal of Evaluation in Clinical Practice* (Vol. 30, Issue 4, pp. 548–558). John Wiley and Sons Inc. https://doi.org/10.1111/jep.13970

Hutcherson, C. A., Seppala, E. M., & Gross, J. J. (2008). Loving-kindness meditation increases social connectedness. *Emotion*, *8*(5), 720–724. https://doi.org/10.1037/a0013237

Jazaieri, H., Jinpa, G. T., McGonigal, K., Rosenberg, E. L., Finkelstein, J., Simon-Thomas, E., Cullen, M., Doty, J. R., Gross, J. J., & Goldin, P. R. (2013). Enhancing compassion: A randomized controlled trial of a compassion cultivation training program. *Journal of Happiness Studies*, *14*(4), 1113–1126. https://doi.org/10.1007/s10902-012-9373-z

Jazaieri, H., McGonigal, K., Jinpa, T., Doty, J. R., Gross, J. J., & Goldin, P. R. (2014). A randomized controlled trial of compassion cultivation training: Effects on mindfulness, affect, and emotion regulation. *Motivation and Emotion*, *38*(1), 23–35. https://doi.org/10.1007/s11031-013-9368-z

Johnson, S. (2018). *The ReMEDI Project: Reverse Mentoring for Equality, Diversity and Inclusion* (pp. 1–35). The University of Nottingham.

Kang, Y., Gray, J. R., & Dovidio, J. F. (2014). The nondiscriminating heart: Lovingkindness meditation training decreases implicit intergroup bias. *Journal of Experimental Psychology: General*, *143*(3), 1306–1313. https://doi.org/10.1037/a0034150

Kauff, M., Bührmann, T., Gölz, F., Simon, L., Lüers, G., van Kampen, S., Kraus de Camargo, O., Snyman, S., & Wulfhorst, B. (2023). Teaching interprofessional collaboration among future healthcare professionals. *Frontiers in Psychology*, *14*. https://doi.org/10.3389/fpsyg.2023.1185730

Kelemen, T. K., Matthews, S. H., Matthews, M. J., & Henry, S. E. (2023). Humble leadership: A review and synthesis of leader expressed humility. In *Journal of Organizational Behavior* (Vol. 44, Issue 2, pp. 202–224). John Wiley and Sons Ltd. https://doi.org/10.1002/job.2608

Klimecki, O. M. (2019). The role of empathy and compassion in conflict resolution. *Emotion Review*, *11*(4), 310–325. https://doi.org/10.1177/1754073919838609

Knox, M. C., & Franco, P. L. (2022). Acceptability and feasibility of an online version of the self-compassion for healthcare communities program. *Psychology, Health & Medicine*, 1–11. https://doi.org/10.1080/13548506.2022.2094428

Kok, B. E., & Singer, T. (2017). Effects of contemplative dyads on engagement and perceived social connectedness over 9 months of mental training a randomized clinical trial. *JAMA Psychiatry, 74*(2), 126–134. https://doi.org/10.1001/jamapsychiatry.2016.3360

Kruse, E., Chancellor, J., Ruberton, P. M., & Lyubomirsky, S. (2014). An upward spiral between gratitude and humility. *Social Psychological and Personality Science, 5*(7), 805–814. https://doi.org/10.1177/1948550614534700

Lehmann, M., Pery, S., Kluger, A. N., Hekman, D. R., Owens, B. P., & Malloy, T. E. (2022). Relationship-specific (dyadic) humility: How your humility predicts my psychological safety and performance. *Journal of Applied Psychology, 108*(5), 809–825. https://doi.org/10.1037/apl0001059

Lown, B. A. (2021). Translational, transformative compassion to support the healthcare workforce. *Journal of Healthcare Management, 66*(4), 254–257. https://doi.org/10.1097/JHM-D-21-00139

Maben, J., Taylor, C., Reynolds, E., McCarthy, I., & Leamy, M. (2021). Realist evaluation of Schwartz rounds® for enhancing the delivery of compassionate healthcare: Understanding how they work, for whom, and in what contexts. *BMC Health Services Research, 21*(1), 1–24. https://doi.org/10.1186/s12913-021-06483-4

Maner, S., & Morris, Paul. G. (2019). A systematic review of the effectiveness of compassion-focused imagery in improving psychological outcomes in clinical and non-clinical adult populations. *Prospero*, 0–2. https://doi.org/10.1002/cpp.2801

McClelland, L. E., & Vogus, T. J. (2021). Infusing, sustaining, and replenishing compassion in health care organizations through compassion practices. *Health Care Management Review, 46*(1), 55–65. https://doi.org/10.1097/HMR.0000000000000240

Michalec, B. (for additional references). (2023). *A researcher's prescription for better health care: A dose of humility for doctors, nurses and clinicians*. https://theconversation.com/a-researchers-prescription-for-better-health-care-a-dose-of-humility-for-doctors-nurses-and-clinicians-210175?utm_source=Receive+News+from+the+John+Templeton+Foundation&utm_campaign=afc5172588-EMAIL_CAMPAIGN_2023_possibilities_20231206&utm_medium=email&utm_term=0_-938f7e3a64-%5BLIST_EMAIL_ID%5D

Michalec, B., Cuddy, M. M., Felix, K., Gur-Arie, R., Tilburt, J. C., & Hafferty, F. W. (2024). Positioning humility within healthcare delivery - From doctors' and nurses' perspectives. *Human Factors in Healthcare, 5*. https://doi.org/10.1016/j.hfh.2023.100061

Neff, K. D., Knox, M. C., Long, P., & Gregory, K. (2020). Caring for others without losing yourself: An adaptation of the mindful self-compassion program for healthcare communities. *Journal of Clinical Psychology, 76*(9), 1543–1562. https://doi.org/10.1002/jclp.23007

Nursing and Midwifery Council. (2018). *The Code. Professional standards of practice and behaviour for nurses, midwives and nursing associates*. www.nmc.org.uk/code

Nutsford, D., Pearson, A. L., Kingham, S., & Reitsma, F. (2016). Residential exposure to visible blue space (but not green space) associated with lower psychological distress in a capital city. *Health and Place, 39*, 70–78. https://doi.org/10.1016/j.healthplace.2016.03.002

Osei-Tutu, K. (2024). Redefining excellence in health care: Uniting inclusive compassion and shared humanity within a transformative physician competency model. *Canadian Medical Association Journal, 196*(11), E381–E383. https://doi.org/10.1503/cmaj.231273

Pavlova, A., Paine, S.-J., Tuato'o, A., & Consedine, N. S. (2024). Healthcare compassion interventions co-design and feasibility inquiry with clinicians and healthcare leaders in Aotearoa/New Zealand. *Social Science & Medicine,* 117327. https://doi.org/10.1016/j.socscimed.2024.117327

Pavlova, A., Wang, C. X. Y., Boggiss, A. L., O'Callaghan, A., & Consedine, N. S. (2022). Predictors of physician compassion, empathy, and related constructs: A systematic review. *Journal of General Internal Medicine, 37*(4), 900–911. https://doi.org/10.1007/s11606-021-07055-2

Porges, S. W. (2022). Polyvagal theory: A science of safety. In *Frontiers in Integrative Neuroscience* (Vol. 16). Frontiers Media S.A. https://doi.org/10.3389/fnint.2022.871227

Raza, A., & Onyesoh, K. (2020). Reverse mentoring for senior NHS leaders: A new type of relationship. *Future Healthcare Journal, 7*(1), 94–96. https://doi.org/10.7861/fhj.2019-0028

Reynolds, C. W., Shen, M. R., Englesbe, M. J., & Kwakye, G. (2023). Humility: A revised definition and techniques for integration into surgical education. *Journal of the American College of Surgeons, 236*(6), 1261–1264. https://doi.org/10.1097/XCS.0000000000000640

Riches, S., Iannelli, H., Reynolds, L., Fisher, H. L., Cross, S., & Attoe, C. (2022). Virtual reality-based training for mental health staff: A novel approach to increase empathy, compassion, and subjective understanding of service user experience. *Advances in Simulation, 7*(1). https://doi.org/10.1186/s41077-022-00217-0

Rodrigues Saturn, S. (2017). Two factors that fuel compassion: The oxytocin system and the social experience of moral elevation. In E. M. Seppala, E. Simon-Thomas, S. L. Brown, M. C. Worline, C. D. Cameron, & J. R. Doty (Eds.), *The Oxford handbook of compassion science* (First edition, pp. 121–131). Oxford University Press.

Schültke, L., Warth, M., Alpers, G. W., Ditzen, B., & Aguilar-Raab, C. (2023). Better together than alone? Investigating dyadic compassion meditation in an experimental study. *Journal of Social and Personal Relationships.* https://doi.org/10.1177/02654075231205452

Sinclair, S., Dhingra, S., Bouchal, S. R., MacInnis, C., Harris, D., Roze des Ordons, A., & Pesut, B. (2024). The initial validation of an evidence-informed, competency-based, Applied Compassion Training (EnACT) program: A multimethod study. *BMC Medical Education, 24*(1). https://doi.org/10.1186/s12909-024-05663-0

Stell, A. J., & Farsides, T. (2016). Brief loving-kindness meditation reduces racial bias, mediated by positive other-regarding emotions. *Motivation and Emotion, 40*(1), 140–147. https://doi.org/10.1007/s11031-015-9514-x

Stellar, J. E., Gordon, A., Anderson, C. L., Piff, P. K., McNeil, G. D., & Keltner, D. (2018). Awe and humility. *Journal of Personality and Social Psychology, 114*(2), 258–269. https://doi.org/10.1037/pspi0000109

Warren, M. A., & Warren, M. T. (2021). The EThIC model of virtue-based allyship development: A new approach to equity and inclusion in organizations. *Journal of Business Ethics, 0123456789*. https://doi.org/10.1007/s10551-021-05002-z

West, M. A. (2021). *Compassionate Leadership*. Swirling Leaf Press.

White, M. P., Alcock, I., Grellier, J., Wheeler, B. W., Hartig, T., Warber, S. L., Bone, A., Depledge, M. H., & Fleming, L. E. (2019). Spending at least 120 minutes a week in nature is associated with good health and wellbeing. *Scientific Reports, 9*(1), 1–11. https://doi.org/10.1038/s41598-019-44097-3

Wilson-Mendenhall, C. D., Dunne, J. D., & Davidson, R. J. (2022). Visualizing compassion: Episodic simulation as contemplative practice. *Mindfulness*. https://doi.org/10.1007/s12671-022-01842-6

Zeng, X., Chiu, C. P. K. K., Wang, R., Oei, T. P. S. S., Leung, F. Y. K., & Simpson, S. G. (2015). The effect of loving-kindness meditation on positive emotions: A meta-analytic review. *Frontiers in Psychology, 6*(November), 1–14. https://doi.org/10.3389/fpsyg.2015.01693

Appendix 1
Web Links Document

Resources for Chapter 11

The Schwartz Center for Compassionate Healthcare (US)
https://www.theschwartzcenter.org

The Point of Care Foundation (UK)
https://www.pointofcarefoundation.org.uk

Professor Kristin Neff's website (US)
https://self-compassion.org

Compassion Institute
https://www.compassioninstitute.com

Professor Paul Gilbert's Compassionate Mind Foundation website (UK)
https://www.compassionatemind.co.uk/resource/resources

The Greater Good Science Center

The Greater Good Science Center (https://greatergood.berkeley.edu) affiliated with the University of Berkeley in California has a searchable catalogue of evidence-based articles and free meditations. Also, those relating directly to compassion for oneself and others, there are a number of other resources on the website that help to support and nurture the capacity for compassion and well-being.

A common humanity meditation to help cultivate compassion for others:
https://ggia.berkeley.edu/practice/common_humanity_meditation

There is a strong relationship between awe and humility and feeling more connected to other people.

An article written by a physician about awe in the context of health-care: https://greatergood.berkeley.edu/article/item/is_awe_a_path_to_resilience_in_caring_professions

Connecting with and re-experiencing a 'compassionate moment' with a patient or colleague in supervision helps to stimulate the oxytocin-opiate-parasympathetic system and the growing embodiment of oneself as a compassionate professional.

An article on how to do this:
https://greatergood.berkeley.edu/article/item/taking_in_the_good

A gratitude and connection meditation:
https://ggia.berkeley.edu/practice/gratitude_meditation

A 13-minute video on the four pillars of well-being, each of which can be cultivated:
https://greatergood.berkeley.edu/video/item/four_constituents_of_well-being

Index

For Product Safety Concerns and Information please contact our EU
representative GPSR@taylorandfrancis.com
Taylor & Francis Verlag GmbH, Kaufingerstraße 24, 80331 München, Germany

www.ingramcontent.com/pod-product-compliance
Lightning Source LLC
Chambersburg PA
CBHW070350270326
41926CB00017B/4071